THE Enchanting ART OF Aromatherapy

For those who wish to harmonise
their environment and health.
Essential oils create mood,
a subtle atmosphere and
a state of consciousness
to every individual's nature.

The knowledge of the pure
essential oils of plants
— remedies that can delight,
inspire and heal.

By *Salvatore Battaglia*

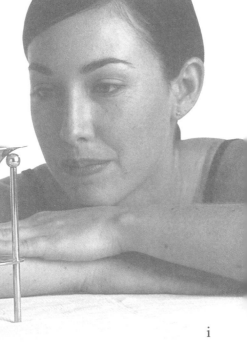

i

Note to Readers

The Enchanting Art of Aromatherapy is concerned with the use of essential oils for a wide range of health problems. Illness, however, can be highly unpredictable and the best possible expertise should always be consulted. The author and publisher accept no liability for any claims arising from the use of any remedy discussed.

If in doubt about using the essential oils please consult a qualified aromatherapist. It must be stressed that a holistic approach to aromatherapy incorporates a healthy diet, lifestyle and general attitude towards life.

Salvatore Battaglia

The Enchanting Art of Aromatherapy.

1st Edition September 1988
2nd Edition April 1991
3rd Edition May 1995
4th Edition June 2003

ISBN 0 7316 4006 3

Published by

The International Centre of Holistic Aromatherapy
P.O Box 635
Albert Street BC Qld, 4002
Phone (07) 3012 8160 Fax (07) 3012 8161
Email info@icha.edu.au
www.icha.edu.au

Designed and typeset by Ingrid van Grysen at Australian Academic Press
Printed in Australia by Watson Ferguson and Company, Brisbane.

Preface to 4th edition

Aromatherapy has now become one of the most sought after natural therapies. What has lead to this meteoric popularity in this ancient but new therapy?

There are many factors that have contributed to aromatherapy's popularity. These include:

- The ease in which essential oils can be incorporated into so many different products, whether they be products to scent the home, skin care products or bath products just to name a few.

- Essential oils are readily available to the general public.

- Aromatherapy is very much associated with a feel good therapy.

- The aesthetic appeal of aromatherapy which involves two senses that are often neglected in today's society, that of touch and smell.

Since *The Enchanting Art of Aromatherapy* was written in 1988, we have come to know much more about olfaction and the pharmacology of essential oils. I have added new sections to the book to include the latest information on olfaction, chemistry and the pharmacology of essential oils. The essential oil profiles have been considerably updated and I have included eight new essential oils.

Salvatore Battaglia
2003

Preface to 3rd edition

It was in 1987 when I first started work on this book, and in the last eight years aromatherapy has blossomed into one of the most popular natural therapies, not only for lay people and natural health practitioners, but also for the medical profession. Many hospitals in the United Kingdom now use aromatherapy and the trend is slowly following in Australia.

While many people are turning to natural therapies, I do stress that aromatherapy, as any other form of natural healing, cannot wave a 'magic wand' and provide a miracle cure. A body which has been abused for years by tobacco, alcohol, junk food, stress, overwork or neglect will not be capable of responding overnight to any kind of natural remedy. True healing takes time and involves changes to lifestyle and attitudes.

I see no harm in essential oil being used as home remedies, provided they are used sensibly and correctly. Essential oils, after all are so much fun to use – they can be used as room fresheners, in baths, in massage and are extremely beneficial as home remedies for many minor ailments.

We must also realise the limitations of self-treatment. Do treat yourself for minor, common ailments, but for long-term, deep-seated problems, seek professional advice. If a problem does not improve seek professional advice.

In this new revised edition, wintergreen has been excluded for safety reasons, the therapeutic section has been expanded, new essential oils and carrier oils have been included and the format of the book has improved to make the book easier to read.

I would like to thank all of you who have supported aromatherapy and my hope is that this book will help to broaden your own horizons just a little.

Salvatore Battaglia
1995

About the Author

Salvatore Battaglia has been passionate about natural therapies for most of his life. He holds qualifications in herbal medicine, natural therapies, acupuncture and aromatherapy.

Together with Carolyn Stubbin, also an accomplished author of the book *Do It Yourself Pure Plant Skin Care*, they established Perfect Potion. Perfect Potion has the reputation of providing the world's finest quality essential oils and pure plant based skin care preparations.

Salvatore's dedication to aromatherapy has seen him hold positions in professional associations and government committees to ensure that the educational standards of professional aromatherapy are maintained and improved.

In 1995, Salvatore wrote *The Complete Guide to Aromatherapy*, which is now internationally recognised as the most authoritive textbook for aromatherapy.

He has been teaching aromatherapy since 1987. In 2000, Salvatore established The International Centre of Holistic Aromatherapy, a government approved training organisation offering the most comprehensive professional aromatherapy training in the world.

Contents

I
Introduction

Aromatherapy has emerged as one of the most popular forms of natural therapy. This is not surprising, considering that it represents a holistic treatment that has become an integral part of a lifestyle for many people.

Whether you are using aromatherapy as a complete natural therapy or simply as a pure luxury, it will be guaranteed to delight the senses, heal the body and uplift the mind.

Introduction

In the western world we tend to take for granted the variety of scents, perfumes, fragrances, aromas, odours and smells we encounter everyday. If we live in or near a city we may encounter nothing more than traces of fuel and chemical fumes that have become a part of our lives. Even inside where we may hope to escape this constant attack on our olfactory senses we often breathe recycled air, frequently tainted by tobacco smoke and many other indiscernible odours on our overworked noses. If we are lucky enough, we hurry home to our little patches of garden in time to inhale the wonderful aroma and freshness of plants, leaves and flowers.

Of course we ensure that our home smells nice, fresh and clean with manufactured scents and fragrances — one squirt and the toilet is filled with pine forests, the bathroom with lilies and the kitchen abounds with lemon. But there is often precious little of the true scent in many of these pleasant contrivances.

Yet thousands of years ago, scholars and healers found that scent of natural oils induced a deep, relaxed respiration. They discovered that different scents produced quite different effects on the nervous system. Offensive smells immediately caused a response of extreme displeasure, while pleasant scents immediately awakened a positive response and a general rejuvenation of the spirits.

Today we can still experience the intense pleasures of nature's most delightful scents. Whether we are by the seaside, out in the country or in the garden, we will pause to breathe deeply so that our deprived olfactory senses enjoy the new sensations and joys. We are momentarily restored to youthful vigour.

If you find it increasingly difficult to achieve this instant rejuvenation, the only alternative is to create your own fragrant atmosphere at home or at work. Aromatherapy can do just that.

Aromatherapy is the gentle science based on the use of essential oils derived from plants. Apart from their pleasing aromas, essential oils are valued for their potent cosmetic and therapeutic values. The essential oils are able to stimulate the body's self healing processes.

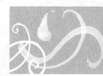

What is Aromatherapy?

The word 'aromatherapy' is often misleading, as it implies that 'aromas' are used therapeutically. While the aromas of essential oils are of therapeutic value, the true value of aromatherapy becomes obvious when we realise the vast range of qualities associated with the essential oils. The definition of aromatherapy that I like to use is:

The use of pure essential oils to seek to influence, to change or modify, mind, body or spirit; physiology or mood.

It is a pleasant therapy, with powerful physiological effects on the body. The essential oils can influence blood pressure, regulate nerve function, aid digestion and have potent anti-bacterial properties. It is also known that essential oils can affect our mental and emotional well being. We respond to smell more emotionally than we respond to other senses, because the olfactory nerves pass directly from the nose to the limbic system, which is the emotional centre of the brain.

History of Aromatherapy

The use of the oils is by no means new. There is much evidence that essential oils were used back in the ancient days of the Egyptians, Greeks and Romans where they were highly regarded for cosmetic and therapeutic uses. During the times of the pharaohs, splendid gardens were stocked with medicinal herbs collected from all over the world. The temple priests and the physicians of the day formulated and prepared medicinal concoctions of essential oils. They also used the essential oils for embalming and for creating perfumes to scent the temples.

Greek physicians visiting Egypt brought back an increased knowledge of the essential oils. Marestheus, a renowned physician, noted that the aromatic plants often possessed stimulating and edifying properties. He discovered that rose and other fruity and spicy scents as being invigorating for the tired mind.

The knights of the Crusades bought back to Europe from the Middle East, aromatic essences and waters, which became so popular that perfumes began to be manufactured. The importance of herbal and aromatic plants was realised when the bubonic plague reached Europe in the 14th century. Fires were ordered in the streets at night, burning aromatic frankincense and pine. Indoors, incense and perfumed candles were burnt to combat infection and disguise the stench of death.

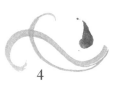

4

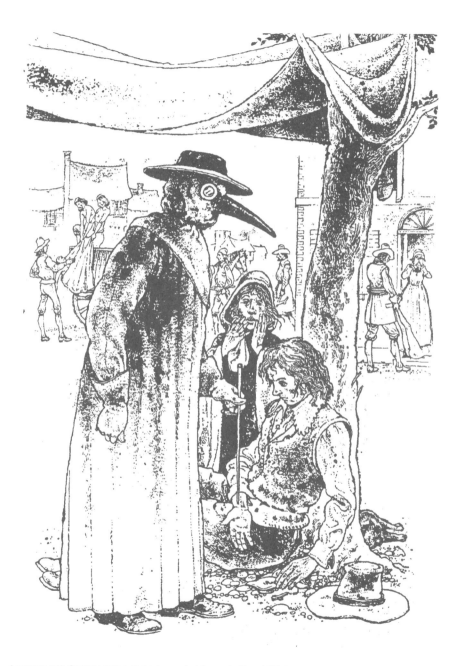

A seventeenth Century plague doctor is wearing the protective clothing
of his profession — a leather gown, leather gloves and a leather mask.
The beak through which he breathes is filled with cinnamon, cloves and
other aromatic herbs. Modern evidence has shown that clove kills the
bacillus that causes typhoid.

While the use of the essential oils dates back thousands of years, it is surprising to know that the term 'aromatherapy' was only coined in the 1930's by a French chemist called R.H. Gattefosse. He is regarded as the father of aromatherapy. In the course of his research, he is said to have burned his hand, to have applied lavender essential oil, and to have found the healing to be remarkably quick. His work revealed that it was possible for the essential oils to penetrate the skin, and be absorbed into the blood stream.

However, it was Marguerite Maury, a French biochemist who extended the study of essential oils outside the medical field to study the absorptive properties of essential oils through the skin. She led the way in the use of essential oils in both beauty therapy and health care, and promoted the use of essential oils by massage. Maury is often attributed as laying down the fundamental principles of holistic aromatherapy today. She emphasised the importance of applying the essential oils externally, diluted in vegetable oil, in combination with massage.

Aromatherapy Today

While natural medicine has become popular with a large segment of the community, the popularity and interest in aromatherapy has been overwhelming. I believe that this is because aromatherapy is 'a feel good therapy' and is so simple to administer and the essential oils add a sense of luxury to the treatment. The essential oils are usually administered by massage, in an oil vaporiser or added to baths.

Aromatherapy is a very pleasant therapy that makes use of two close range senses — that of touch and smell. Some essential oils have anti-bacterial properties, others have psychotherapeutic benefits, relieving stress, depression and insomnia.

When I speak to clients who have come for an aromatherapy treatment, I find that they are drawn to its multifaceted aspect of aromatherapy which combines practical hands-on skills, natural fragrant essential oils and a holistic caring approach. Holistic aromatherapy means using the essential oils to facilitate the natural healing process of the body.

The overall aim of holistic aromatherapy is to bring about a state of harmony and balance within the body, mind and soul. Holistic aromatherapy ensure that the essential oils work on the:

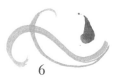

- **Body** — via the pharmacological actions of the essential oils. For example, the expectorant and decongestant activity of eucalyptus essential oil can be directly traced to the 1,8-cineole content, which has the property of reducing the swelling of mucous membranes and of loosening phlegm.

- **Mind** — via the psychotherapeutic actions of the essential oils. Researchers are discovering more and more about the elusive connection between our sense of smell and the emotional and behavioural centres of our brain.

- **Soul** — via the metaphysical actions of the essential oils. Essential oils have a wonderfully rich history of use in religious and mediative ceremonies of the ancient Egyptians, Indians and Romans. Many people still make use of fragrance in their pursuit for higher enlightenment through meditation, chakra balancing and psychic healing.

What are Essential Oils?

Essential oils are natural plant extracts that occur widely in the plant kingdom, not only in the flowers, leaves and fruit but also in the roots, stems and in other parts of the plants. The essential oils are usually secreted from special glands, ducts or cells in one or several parts of aromatic plants and from the sap and tissue of certain trees. It is the essential oil that gives the plant its distinctive aroma. Crush a leaf of eucalyptus or fresh basil or peppermint, and notice how strongly the aroma penetrates your fingers and fills the air around you.

The cost of the essential oil is usually proportional to the amount of oil glands or ducts present in the plant. Oils from plants with few glands or ducts are more costly.

For example did you know that:
- 100kg of eucalyptus are needed to yield 10 litres of oil?
- 100kg of lavender flowers are needed to yield 3 litres of oil?
- 100kg of roses are needed to yield 100mls of oil?

Most flowers, seeds, barks, roots, resins, leaves and woods contain essential oil, usually in rather minute quantities. Essential oils are extracted from different parts of the plants.

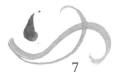

Examples of the distribution of essential oils in plants are:

Flower:	jasmine, neroli, rose, ylang ylang.
Flowering tops & leaves:	rosemary, lavender, peppermint, basil.
Leaves:	patchouli, petitgrain, eucalyptus, pine, tea tree.
Fruit rind:	grapefruit, sweet orange, mandarin, lemon, lime.
Seeds:	aniseed, black pepper, cardamom, fennel.
Berries:	juniper, may chang.
Resin:	frankincense, myrrh.
Wood:	Virginian and Atlas cedarwood, rosewood, sandalwood.
Roots:	ginger, vetiver.

Sometimes several essential oils can be extracted from the same plant. The bitter orange tree for example, contains bitter orange essential oil from the rind of the fruits, petitgrain oil from the leaves and neroli oil from the flowers. Each of these essential oils has a distinct smell with different therapeutic properties.

Essential oils are odorous and highly volatile, evaporating readily in open air. They are different from vegetables oils in that they have a consistency more like water rather than vegetable oil.

How are Essential Oils Extracted?

Essential oils can be extracted from the plants in a number of ways. The most common and modern method used today is steam distillation. This involves placing the plant material in a still and passing steam through it. The essential oil evaporates along with the water. The distillate is then cooled and the essential oil which is not water-soluble is easily separated from the water.

Distillation is a very simple method of processing large quantities of plant matter in a relatively short time. The only disadvantage is that essential oils are often liable to modification because of the heat involved.

The essential oils from citrus fruits such as orange, lemon, bergamot and mandarin are found in the rind and are obtained by a simple process known as cold pressed expression. Once carried out by hand, by squeezing the essential oil from the rind, machines using centrifugal force have now replaced this technique.

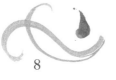

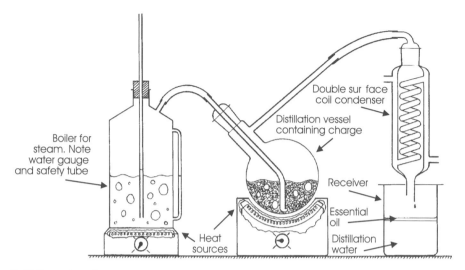

Distillation equipment

Enfleurage was once a common method of extracting essential oils. This involves the use of animal fat, usually lard, to absorb the essential oil, which is then separated out using alcohol. The evaporation of the alcohol then leaves behind the essential oil. Enfleurage is rarely used today, with the exception of jasmine and tuberose. This highly labour-intensive and time-consuming enfleurage method has led to the development and use of solvent extraction methods.

Extraction with solvents involves a complicated series of extractors producing a mixture of odoriferous materials together with natural plant waxes, known as a concrete. The next stage involves the mixture being dissolved in alcohol, before being distilled to produce the most concentrated oil, known as an absolute. Solvent extracted oils are generally referred to as absolutes.

A more recent method of extracting essential oil involves the use of low temperature, high pressure carbon dioxide. An extremely high quality essential oil is produced by this method. However it is an extremely expensive technique because of the very high pressure that is required. At this stage there are relatively few essential oils available by this method.

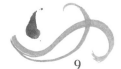

Buying Quality Essential Oils

The essential oil industry is very large, catering to the needs of the food flavouring, perfumery, pharmaceutical and aromatherapy industries. The standard of essential oils produced for the perfumery or for food flavouring, however, are not necessarily suitable for use in aromatherapy.

Whether for professional or home aromatherapy use, the essential oils used should be of the highest quality. The aromatherapy industry has established its own criteria for quality of essential oils used for therapeutic applications. Essential oils must be 'pure and natural' and 'genuine and authentic'. To ensure this the following information should be specified:

- the botanical name of the plant from which the oil is extracted.
- the part of plant from which the oil is extracted.
- the extraction method used.
- the country of origin.

Cost is also used as an indication of quality. If the essential oil is very inexpensive, check to see whether it has been diluted with a carrier oil or if it is a reconstituted or synthetic oil. Buy from a well-known, reputable supplier, preferably one who specialises in aromatherapy.

The Botanical Name

Many herbs have the same common name and this may lead to an oversight and subsequent mistakes. For example, when using chamomile oil it is important to identify whether Roman or German chamomile is preferred. The two oils are quite distinct. German chamomile oil, a rich inky blue oil produced from *Matricaria recutita*, is rich in sesquiterpenes which give the oil its excellent anti-inflammatory properties. On the other hand, Roman chamomile, a pale yellow oil produced from *Anthemis nobilis*, is rich in esters which are responsible for the oil's antispasmodic and sedative properties.

There are several species of lavender. Spike lavender, produced from *Lavendula spika* is naturally rich in camphor and cineole, this makes it useful as an inhalation for respiratory infections and for soothing muscular aches and pains. On the other hand true lavender, distilled from *Lavendula angustifolia* is rich in linalool and linalyl acetate and is typically used in aromatherapy for relaxation and skin care.

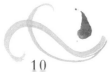

The Part of the Plant Used

Different parts of the plant will produce essential oils of varying qualities, characteristics and aroma. For example, the bitter orange tree is a classic example of a tree from which many essential oils are produced; neroli oil from the flowers, petitgrain oil from the leaves and bitter orange oil from the rind. Each of these essential oils have their own unique properties.

Method of Extraction

Often an essential oil may be produced by more than one process of extraction, thus yielding essential oils of different chemical composition and quality. For example, it is possible to obtain distilled lime oil and cold pressed lime oil.

Rose oil is either produced by solvent extraction, known as rose absolute, or rose otto produced by distillation. The rich, heavy floral aroma of rose absolute is described as being sensual and exotic while the delicate floral aroma of rose otto is soothing and calming.

Country of Origin

Often an essential oil from a particular area is of superior quality. The oil becomes known by the area it which it is grown. For example, French lavender or Tasmanian lavender. Even though both essential oils are distilled from *Lavendula angustifolia*, they have different characteristics which may be due to the environment, cultivation practices and the genetics of the plant stocks.

Natural Versus Synthetic

In recent years there has been much confusion between pure essential oils and fragrance oils, which are nothing more than synthetic fragrances, ideal for perfumery and pot pourris.

For example, it will take more than one tonne of rose petals to produce 1kg of rose oil. Most of the rose oil found on store shelves almost invariably is synthetic. Given this situation and the high demand for essential oils in perfumery it is not surprising that chemical research has succeeded in producing rather good imitations of these oils. While these products smell very nice, it needs to be emphasised that the synthetic oils do not have any therapeutic qualities of the essential oil.

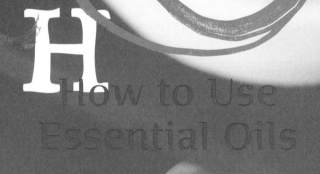

How to Use
Essential Oils

One of the best aspects of aromatherapy is the diversity with which the essential oils can be used. Essential oils can be incorporated into your daily routine, without requiring complicated adjustments to your lifestyle.

This chapter describes the various techniques in which essential oils may be used.

How to Use Essential Oils

There are various ways in which essential oils can be used to alleviate many health problems and create a sense of well being:

- Inhalation
- Massage
- Compress
- Bath

Through massage the essential oils are easily absorbed into the body through the skin. Direct inhalation is also very effective whether it be simply sniffing the oil from the bottle or using an oil vaporiser. Baths are very effective as the essential oils are absorbed through the skin as well as being inhaled.

Some aromatherapists and doctors in France recommend internal ingestion of the essential oils. Excellent as essential oils are, I advise people against taking essential oils internally, as the essential oils are highly concentrated and may cause irritation of the gastro-intestinal tract. In France, the medical doctors prescribing essential oils often ensure that the essential oils are encapsulated to avoid irritation of the gastro-intestinal tract.

Inhalations

Inhalations are mainly used for the treatment of stress, headaches and respiratory tract problems such as asthma, colds, sore throats, blocked sinuses and coughs.

One of the easiest ways to inhale essential oils is to simply place about 10 drops on a tissue or handkerchief and inhale the aroma as often as possible. Place the handkerchief next to your pillow at night beside your nose, to ensure a free breathing passage during the night. Another way of clearing stuffy head colds is by inhaling the essential oil through a steam inhaler.
Add about 10 drops of oil to 100mls of hot water. It is best to place a towel over your head and the basin.

An oil vaporiser is another popular method to help you create the ideal ambience in your home or workplace. Nowadays we have quite a selection of vaporisers to choose from, whether

it is a candle style or electric powered. Carefully follow the instructions provided by the manufacture before using your vaporiser.

Most candle vaporisers will require you to place a small quantity of water in the small dish on top of the oil vaporiser, then add 5 to 10 drops of your selected essential oil or a blend of essential oils. You then light the candle and keep it alight for approximately 30 minutes. Take care that the water and essential oil in the dish does not completely evaporate before blowing out the candle.

Baths

Since the days of antiquity, aromatic baths have been used to relax and revitalise. For a full body bath, use 5–10 drops of the appropriate essential oil in a tub of warm water. To ensure that the essential oil disperses in the water use a dispersant. A dispersant is usually a vegetable oil derived product that allows the essential oil to dissolve in water. Add 5 drops of essential oil to each 10ml of dispersant, and then add 5ml of the blended dispersant to a tub of water. Foot or hand baths may also be prepared by adding 5 drops of essential oil to a bowl of warm water.

Enjoy approximately 15 minutes soaking in the fragrant bath, taking deep inhalations of the pleasant aromas to relax your mind and nervous system, while your skin absorbs the natural healing oils.

Conditions that can benefit from baths are insomnia, nervous tension, muscular disorders, circulatory problems, menstrual problems, headaches and fluid retention.

Try some of these wonderful bath recipes:

Winter Bath — *to help ward off colds and stimulate circulation*

ginger	2 drops
eucalyptus, blue mallee	3 drops
tea tree	2 drops
lemon	2 drops
dispersing bath oil	10ml

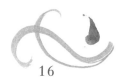

Sunrise Bath — *perfect way to start the day*

rosemary	2 drops
juniper berry	3 drops
ginger	3 drops
dispersing bath oil	10ml

Lemon Zest Bath — *revitalising and energising*

sweet orange	4 drops
lemon	4 drops
dispersing bath oil	10ml

Relaxing Bath — *soothing and relaxing*

lavender	3 drops
sandalwood	3 drops
ylang ylang	2 drops
dispersing bath oil	10ml

Refreshing Bath — *great for those hot summer days*

peppermint	2 drops
lime, distilled	3 drops
lavender	2 drops
dispersing bath oil	10ml

Detoxifying Bath — *purifying and detoxifying*

juniper berry	2 drops
grapefruit	3 drops
fennel seed	2 drops
dispersing bath oil	10ml

Foot and Hand Baths

A foot or hand bath is a simple way of treating yourself while sitting down at night. All that is needed is a bowl of hot water and 10 drops of essential oil. Steep the hands or feet for 10 to 15 minutes. Wrap the hands or feet in a dry towel after soaking. Conditions such as arthritis, rheumatism, dermatitis, dry skin and fluid retention are best treated by this method.

Massage

Massage is perhaps the oldest and simplest of all medical treatments. It can be described as the art of touching. Massage is a two-way flow of touch and response, a mutual exchange of energy. Through your hands you perceive and discover the uniqueness of the person you are touching; through their skin they are receiving the gift of your touch, the caring contact and movement.

Massage is not only physical, it has a psychological benefit. One advantage of massage is that it is as pleasant to give as much as it is to receive. Massage can be stimulating or soothing, depending upon the speed, rhythm and depth of the strokes. It can make a person feel alert and ready to run a marathon, or conversely, relaxed and sleepy. It can relieve tension, soothe away headaches, relax taunt and aching muscles and banish insomnia.

Care and sensitivity, a little time and energy, and a good pair of hands are all that is needed to practise massage. Before you begin, ensure that the environment and surroundings are pleasant and that the room is warm. Comfort is a priority.

Important to the success of massage is your state of mind and attitude to your partner. You should regard each session as a new experience and bring to each person a feeling of genuine care, consideration and respect.

In general, discourage chatting — it will only distract your concentration. Never attempt to massage if you are feeling upset, angry, or not well — not only will your energy be depleted, but your mood will also affect your partner.

It is important to stay centred and give your partner full attention. Many of us spend our lives idly worrying about the future but miss out in the present moment. It is essential to keep your attention on the present, for healing energy transmitted through your hands will be weakened by an absent mind. When you are centred, your intuition guides you and you easily sense your partner's sources of tension and energy imbalances.

How to Use Essential Oils in Massage

For massage purposes, essential oils are usually diluted in a carrier oil. The standard carrier oil used is a vegetable oil. There is no preferred vegetable oil. The selection of the base used is dependent on the benefits of the carrier oil and the cost of the carrier oil.

For example, someone with dry skin would benefit from cold pressed avocado oil, someone with mature skin would benefit from cold pressed rosehip oil and wheatgerm oil, while someone with sensitive skin would benefit from jojoba and evening primrose being used as a base oil.

The recommended dilution rate used is a 1% to 3% dilution of the appropriate essential oil to the carrier oil.

A general rule of thumb is that 1ml of essential oil is approximately 20 drops. This is only an estimate as it will obviously depend on the size of the eye dropper or dripulator and the specific gravity of the essential oil.

If you are preparing a 3% dilution massage blend:

- to 100ml of carrier oil, you add 3ml of essential oil, or 60 drops.
- to 50ml of carrier oil, you add 1.5ml of essential oil, or 30 drops.

If you are using more than one essential oil to make your massage oil, it must be emphasized that the dilution refers to the total combination of essential oils.

When working with babies, children, pregnant women, elderly and persons with sensitive skin you should only use 0.5% to 1.0% dilution.

If you are preparing a 1% dilution massage blend:

- to 100ml of carrier oil, you add 1ml of essential oil, or 20 drops.
- to 50ml of carrier oil, you add 0.5ml of essential oil, or 10 drops.

Conditions that respond to massage include circulatory problems, digestive problems, fluid retention, headaches, insomnia, menstrual problems, musculoskeletal disorders and nervous tension.

Compress

A compress is water and essential oils or herbs applied externally to the body with a cloth. Compresses can be hot or cold, depending on the condition. A hot compress should be as hot as tolerable and a cold compress should have ice in it. Hot compresses are very useful for rheumatic and muscular aches and pain, to relieve menstrual cramping and for drawing out boils. Compresses are commonly used to treat sprains, swellings and headaches. Alternating warm and cold compresses may be used to help speed healing in pulled muscles, sprained ligaments and bruises.

Use 5 drops of essential oil in 200ml of water. Place a cloth, un-medicated gauze or cotton wool into the water, wring out and then cover the area being treated. Place a plastic wrap around the compress and then a towel or blanket on top. Leave the compress on for several hours.

Skin Care Applications

Essential oils can be easily incorporated into a range of skin care preparations.

Emulsions

Creams and lotions are light oil preparations emulsified in water. They may be used to treat most skin conditions or any condition where a massage oil can be used. The benefits of using creams and lotions are that they protect and heal the skin, soothe and moisturise and that they do not leave an oily feeling on the skin.

The basic ingredients needed to make emulsions are emulsifying waxes, water, emollients such as vegetable oils, preservatives and essential oils.

A simple recipe for making a cream is as follows:

emulsifying wax	20gm
coconut	20ml
sweet almond	40ml
purified water	90ml
citrus seed extract	1ml

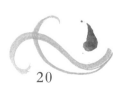

Melt the wax in a bain-marie and stir in the vegetable oils. Bring the water to the same temperature in a separate bowl and add the citrus seed extract. Remove both bowls from the heat and slowly stir the water into the wax mixture. Continue stirring until the mixture cools, then add 1–3% essential oil and store in a jar.

Ointments

An ointment is an oil or fat extraction applied to the skin by rubbing.
It is often called a 'salve' or 'ungent'. It has protective, healing, soothing
and moistening properties. Some examples of ointments include:

- For the treatment of boils, sores, infected cuts and fungal skin conditions
  a soothing and antiseptic ointment can be made using tea tree oil
  and infused calendula oil.
- The rubefacient and analgesic properties of black pepper, ginger, cinnamon
  and peppermint can be used in an ointment to treat arthritis and sports
  injuries. Use before an event to keep the muscles warm and prevent injuries.
- To moisten, soothe and protect dry, irritated skin conditions such as eczema,
  dry chapped skin or lips, use infused calendula oil, infused carrot oil, myrrh
  and German chamomile in an ointment.

For an ointment base, various types of fats such as cocoa butter, shea butter
or lanolin can be used. An ointment can also be made by blending
10% beeswax with 90% vegetable oil such as almond oil.

The amount of essential oil that you would add to an ointment depends
on the purpose of the ointment. If the ointment was for eczema or any
inflammatory skin condition then you would use 1% or less essential oil.
However, an ointment for muscular aches and pain or arthritis can contain
as much as 20% essential oil!

Gels

Gel preparations are used to hydrate, soothe and cool the skin. Gels make
an excellent base for essential oils when a vegetable oil base is not desired.
Gels can be made from plant materials such as linseeds, pectin from citrus peel,
guar gum or xanthan gum. Gels can be used as moisturisers, masks, treatments
for skin problems such as acne and blemished skin and in hair styling products.

The amount of essential oil added to a gel based preparation is usually
0.5% or less.

Masks

Masks can be made from clays, fruit or gels and are used for cleansing the skin
— to absorb excess oil, remove dead skin cells, soften
blackheads, heal damaged and blemished skin, stimulate
circulation in the skin and stimulate healthy cell
regeneration, nourish and moisturise the skin and improve

tone and colour of the skin. The amount of essential oil added to a mask is usually 0.5% or less.

Spritzers

Spritzers can be used for room fresheners, body sprays, non-alcoholic perfumes, insect repellents and deodorants. A spritzer is made by dispersing an essential oil in water and placing the solution into a spray bottle. To do this you will need to obtain an essential oil solubiliser or dispersant and follow the supplier's instructions for dispersing essential oils.

Many books suggest adding the essential oils into water without a solubiliser or dispersant and shaking the bottle before use. This is not an effective or safe way to use the essential oils as a spritzer, especially if it is for topical application. The amount of essential oil added to a spritzer is usually 1% or less.

Safety Issues

It is important to point out that because essential oils are natural substances it does not automatically mean that they are safe. A number of hazards do exist and users of essential oils are most likely to do harm through ignorance of these hazards. As long as the following guidelines are observed aromatherapy will be considered safe.

- Do not apply the pure essential oil directly onto the skin or take internally unless advised by a qualified practitioner.
- Never exceed the recommended dosages.
- Do not use the same oil all the time. For maximum benefit use a blend of oils or alternate the essential oils from week to week.
- Use less than the recommended dilution when making massage oil blends for children and people with sensitive skin. Use only a 1% dilution, i.e. 2 drops to every 10ml of carrier oil.

Contra-indications

Epilepsy

Many aromatherapists consider it sensible for persons with epilepsy to avoid the use of hyssop, rosemary and sage.

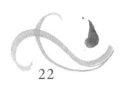

Pregnancy

Many aromatherapists consider it sensible to avoid the use of basil, clary sage, cypress, sweet and bitter fennel, hyssop, juniper berry, sweet marjoram, myrrh, nutmeg, pennyroyal, peppermint, rosemary, sage and thyme during pregnancy.

High Blood Pressure

Many aromatherapists consider it sensible for persons with hypertension to avoid the use of hyssop, rosemary, thyme and sage.

Photosensitivity

Some essential oils such as bergamot, cold pressed lime, bitter orange and lemon may cause the skin to burn when exposed to strong ultra-violet light from sunlight or from a sun bed.

Skin Irritations

Essential oils such as basil, lemon, cinnamon leaf and bark, clove, lemongrass, thyme and tea tree may cause skin irritation to people with sensitive skin. Sensitivity varies from person to person and from oil to oil.

Caring for Essential Oils

Correct storage of essential oils is important. As essential oils are highly volatile and evaporate easily, they should be kept in dark glass bottles at temperatures no higher than 30°C. They should be kept in well-sealed bottles and protected from heat and light. For safety purposes the essential oil bottles should also have a restrictive flow device
and a tamper evident cap.

If stored correctly, most essential oils, will keep for many years. However, citrus oils should be used within two years. For safety purposes ensure that the essential oils that you purchase clearly indicate a 'best used by' or 'expiry date'. Aged essential oils are more likely to have undergone oxidation, hence are more likely to cause dermal irritation.

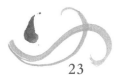

How Does Aromatherapy Work?

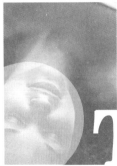
There are a plethora
of self-help aromatherapy books
extolling the virtues of essential oils.
However, when one searches for research
on aromatherapy in scientific publications
and databases, very little is found.

While this may not be such a great
concern for many of us that use essential
oils and have found them beneficial, it has
been said that if the aromatherapy profession
wants to be respected and acknowledged
by the conventional Western medical world,
then it needs to show substantial
and replicable clinical evidence to
support the therapeutic claims made.

How Does Aromatherapy Work?

In search of clinical evidence, researchers and some aromatherapists have turned to pharmacology.
In pharmacology, nature is effectively disintegrated so that the actions of isolated essential oil constituents on isolated areas or functions of the body can be observed as precisely as is possible in a variable world. These observations are then stuck together to make a jigsaw picture of the effect of that substance on the body. It is on this basis that drugs are tested and given to real people. Is this a feasible proposition for determining the pharmacological activity of essential oils?

Many argue that the pharmacological model is too restrictive, focusing only on the physiological influences of the essential oils. The point is that essential oils are chemically complex, and the whole essential oil will have different properties from that of any single constituent. Most pharmacological studies tend to use individual essential oil constituents rather than the whole essential oil. It also does not take into account the dynamic nature of the essential oils, which work on an emotional, mental and spiritual plane.

If the focus of the essential oil's therapeutic properties is based entirely on its chemistry, there is also a concern that legislators may ask for the essential oils to become standardised. This has already happened with Eucalyptus B.P. It is a rectified to ensure that it has at least 75% 1,8-cineole. While 1,8-cineole is identified as an expectorant, it is the higher boiling point residues of eucalyptus, which are removed in the redistillation process that have been identified as having greater antimicrobial properties.

How Essential Oils Enter the Body

Essential oils follow three main pathways to gain entry into the body:

- Ingestion
- Inhalation
- Absorption through the skin

Ingestion is the main medical approach used by doctors in France, but it is not commonly used by aromatherapists in Australia. Unless the aromatherapist has had similar training to the French doctors in the areas of essential oil pharmacology and pathophysiology, I would strongly advise against ingestion.

Inhalation is a very effective route in the treatment of emotional problems such as stress, anxiety and depression. This is because the olfactory nerves in the nose have direct contact with the brain via the limbic system which we shall discuss shortly.

The most common method of utilising essential oils is massage. The skin is considered to be relatively permeable to essential oils. A recent study involving lavender oil diluted in peanut oil massaged over the stomach area for 10 minutes indicated that traces of linalool and linalyl acetate, two of the major components found in lavender, were detected in the blood stream after 20 minutes. After 90 minutes most of the components had been eliminated from the blood.

Once essential oil constituents have passed the epidermis of the skin, usually via the stratum corneum or the sweat glands and the hair follicles, they can be absorbed into the blood capillaries found in the dermis before they are carried away in the circulation.

Chemistry of Essential Oils

In order to gain an understanding of the possible pharmacological properties of essential oils it is necessary to understand the chemistry of essential oils. A knowledge of the chemical composition of essential oils will also assist us in identifying potential hazards and help us in determining the purity of the essential oils.

Almost all of the molecules found in essential oils are composed of carbon, hydrogen and oxygen atoms. The main groups of molecules found in essential oils are terpenes, terpenoid compounds and phenyl propane derived molecules. There are

many other compounds in plants that do not find their way into the essential oil. Among them are all the molecules that are soluble in water, like acids and sugars and molecules such as tannins, flavonoids and carotenoids which are too large to evaporate with the steam distillation.

The molecules found in essential oils may be classified according to their molecular structure. Research by French doctors, Franchomme and Penoel found that the pharmacology of the essential oils can be attributed to the type of molecule found in the oil.

The main groups of molecules found in essential oils are monoterpene hydrocarbons, monoterpene alcohols, sesquiterpenes, phenols, phenyl propane derivatives, ketones, esters, aldehydes and oxides.

Monoterpene Hydrocarbons

Essential oils extracted from citrus peels such as sweet orange, lemon and grapefruit and needle trees such as cypress and pine are rich in monoterpene hydrocarbons.

Monoterpene hydrocarbons have pronounced antiseptic and antiviral effects. However, they oxidise rapidly and tend to exhibit a drying affect on the skin, hence they may be slightly irritating to persons with sensitive skin.

Monoterpene Alcohols

Essential oils such as lavender, rosewood, petitgrain and tea tree are rich in monoterpene alcohols. Monoterpene alcohols generally have antibacterial, antifungal and antiviral properties, and are considered to be the safest and most beneficial of all essential constituents.

Sesquiterpenes

Essential oils such as German chamomile, everlasting and sandalwood are rich in sesquiterpene compounds. Extensive research into sesquiterpene compounds has found them to have excellent anti-inflammatory and anti-allergenic properties. Hence these oils are used in skin care for persons with sensitive skin.

Phenols

Essential oils such as thyme and origano owe their antiseptic and germicidal properties to their phenolic content. However, these essential oils should be used with caution as phenols are highly reactive molecules and are irritating to the skin.

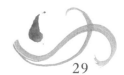

Phenyl Propane Derivatives

Essential oils such as basil, fennel and aniseed have been traditionally used for digestive complaints. The phenol propane derivatives found in these oils contribute to their antispasmodic properties, thus making them useful for treating digestive complaints.

Some essential oils containing phenyl propane derivatives have been labelled as toxic oils. Safrole found in sassafras (now a banned essential oil) and methyl chavicol found in Comoros Island basil, have been found to be potentially carcinogenic while myristicin found in nutmeg and apiol found in parsley seed are neurotoxic.

Ketones

Essential oils rich in ketones are important in aromatherapy because of their ability to ease or increase the flow of mucous and their wound healing properties.

Ketones found in aniseed, fennel and *Eucalyptus dives* are well known for their ability to ease respiratory congestion because of their mucolytic properties. There is a certain level of concern regarding the safety of ketones. Thujone found in wormwood is well known for its neurotoxicity while pulegone found in pennyroyal is hepatotoxic and may be abortifacient.

Esters

Esters found in essential oils generally have a fruity and fragrant odour and tend to be used extensively in perfumery. They are well known for their antispasmodic and sedative properties.

Roman chamomile, clary sage and ylang ylang are examples of essential oils rich in esters and they are well known for their antispasmodic and sedative properties.

Aldehydes

Essential oils rich in aldehydes include lemongrass, may chang and a relatively new Australian essential oil — lemon myrtle. Aldehydes are well known for their antiseptic properties, however they tend to be very unstable and readily oxidise. It is not surprising to note that essential oils rich in aldehydes can be dermal irritants.

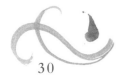

Oxides

Essential oils such as eucalyptus, cajeput and rosemary are rich in 1,8-cineole, an oxide. Essential oils rich in oxides are well known for their expectorant properties and are used in inhalations and topical applications for the treatment of colds, flu, sinusitis and bronchitis.

The main groups of molecules typically found in essential oils

Properties of Essential Oils

Antimicrobial

The term antimicrobial loosely describes the more specific terms; antibacterial, antiviral and antifungal. Generally essential oils rich in monoterpene hydrocarbons, phenols, aldehydes and monoterpene alcohols have excellent antimicrobial properties.

Analgesic

Essential oils with anti-inflammatory properties and circulatory stimulating effects tend to possess analgesic properties. Eugenol found in clove essential oil is well known for its analgesic effect. It is well known for its ability to impart temporary relief from a toothache. Eugenol like other phenols, acts to depress sensory receptors involved in pain perception.

The anti-inflammatory and analgesic properties of methyl salycilate found in wintergreen has traditionally been used in rubs for muscular pain. Menthol found in peppermint has long been employed for the relief of headaches.

Anti-inflammatory

There are a number of essential oils that have been scientifically proven to have anti-inflammatory properties. There are a number of mechanisms believed to be responsible for the anti-inflammatory property of essential oils, such as the ability of some essential oils to inhibit prostaglandins, which are the mediators of inflammation or the ability to improve local circulation. It is known that the beginning of a local inflammation is caused by the contraction of the arteries due to the release of adrenalin.

The anti-inflammatory properties of German chamomile oil are well documented when used topically. German chamomile is considered an anti-inflammatory due to its chamazulene and the α-bisabolol content.

Carminative and Cholagogue

The term carminative is used to describe the removal of gases that have accumulated in the stomach and intestines. Essential oils such as German and Roman chamomile, peppermint, fennel and aniseed have carminative properties.

Generally essential oils which are carminatives have a spasmolytic effect and a cholagogue effect. Essential oils that are cholagogues increase the production of bile. Essential oils such as German chamomile, fennel, grapefruit and rosemary are known to have cholagogue properties.

Detoxifying

Detoxifiers are also known as blood purifiers. The concept of blood purification is difficult for a person with a medical or pharmacological background to understand or agree with. Detoxifying essential oils assist the body's natural eliminatory response by stimulating the liver, lungs, lymphatic system, kidneys, bowels and sweat glands. Any essential oils which has one or more of the following properties is classified as an detoxifier:

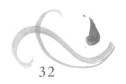

Lymphatic	— assisting the tissue cleaning action of the lymphatic system.
Diaphoretic	— promoting sweating, thus assisting the excretory functions of the skin.
Expectorant	— promoting expulsion of mucus, thus assisting the respiratory system.
Diuretic	— promoting urination, thus assisting the kidneys.
Hepatic	— enhancing liver function, thus assisting the liver's detoxifying function.
Laxative	— promoting bowel movement, thus assisting with the excretory functions of the large intestine.
Emmenagogue	— promoting menstruation, thus assisting in the elimination of menstrual blood.

All of the above properties will help promote detoxification for the general treatment of toxaemia.

Wound Healing

Essential oils have traditionally been used to promote the healing of wounds. Perhaps the most notable story is how Rene Gattefosse burnt his hand in a laboratory explosion and utilised pure lavender oil to heal his wound. He observed the rapid healing and pain relieving effects of lavender.

Other essential oils with wound healing properties include everlasting, frankincense, myrrh, tea tree and yarrow.

Calendula officinalis has been traditionally used for the treatment of skin ailments and to facilitate wound healing. While calendula is not available as a steam distilled essential oil, either an infused oil or an aqueous extract of calendula flowers may be used.

Rosehip vegetable oil is a rich source of polyunsaturated fatty acids, linoleic and linolenic acid. Recent research indicates that topically applied oils containing essential fatty acids will speed the wound healing process by assisting the formation of prostaglandins. Prostaglandins may be involved in the wound healing process by increasing local blood supply, mediating leucocyte emigration into the wound and assisting the synthesis of granulation tissue.

Expectorant and Mucolytic

Essential oils that are expectorants and mucolytic liquefy viscous sputum so it can be easily cleared by coughing. Expectoration is effected by fine hairs (cilia) of the ciliated epithelium lining the respiratory passages, which push the mucus in waves outwards. If the viscosity of the sputum is reduced, the expulsion of the secretions produced by the bronchi becomes easier.

The oxide, 1,8-cineole, which is found in eucalyptus oil is well known for its expectorant properties. It has been postulated that eucalyptus oil has the effect of reducing surface tension between water and air in the lungs, a property which would presumably enhance the effect of the lungs' own surfactant.

Essential oils with expectorant and mucolytic properties such as aniseed, eucalyptus, cajeput, fennel, myrtle, pine, rosemary and thyme are very effective in relieving coughs and mucous congestion.

Nervines

Nervines strengthen and tone the activity of the nervous system. They can actually be stimulants or sedatives. Many nervines are also antispasmodics or relaxants. These essential oils relax the whole body, not only mentally, but also in terms of visceral neuromuscular function.

Relaxants are indicated whenever it is desired to reduce the effects of tension or overactivity of a body system. Therefore in cases of nervous indigestion, bowel problems, bronchial spasms, menstrual spasms and any other physiological disorder where tissue tension is elicited, relaxant essential oils will be beneficial.

Essential oils with relaxant nervine properties include bergamot, German and Roman chamomile, clary sage, geranium, jasmine, lavender, neroli, sweet marjoram, sandalwood and ylang ylang.

Essential oils with stimulant nervine properties include basil, black pepper, cardamom, cinnamon, clove, fennel, ginger, lemon, nutmeg, peppermint, pine, rosemary and thyme.

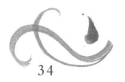

Olfaction

The effect of smell has a powerful influence on the central nervous system. Olfactory researchers are discovering that smell can influence mood, evoke emotions, counteract stress and reduce high blood pressure. To explain how essential oils can affect us in this way we must explore the connection between the sense of smell and the brain.

Essential oils are made up of hundreds of aromatic molecules that are volatile. The essential oil is capable of entering a gaseous state so that it can enter our nose when we inhale. Located at the top of the nasal cavity is the olfactory epithelium which is covered with a thin layer of mucus. Once in the nose, the aromatic molecules migrate through the mucus to the underlying tissue of approximately 10 million olfactory nerve cells. Each olfactory nerve carries a bundle of tiny cilia that are equipped with different receptor cells to fit each aromatic molecule shape, like a key in a lock. The human nose can detect up to 10,000 different odours at very low concentrations.

Smell is the only sense in which the receptor nerve endings are in direct contact with the outside world. It is also interesting to note that the olfactory nerve cells are the only type of nerve cell in the body that can repair itself when damaged.

The olfactory receptors are responsible for converting the odour molecule into an electrical nerve impulse before transmitting it to the olfactory bulb. It is in the olfactory bulb that the electrical nerve impulse is initially processed. The olfactory messages are then sent, via the olfactory tract to the higher olfactory areas of the brain.

From the olfactory bulb two main pathways have been identified. One is the thalamus which then projects to the neocortex in the orbito-frontal cortical region of the brain, and the other is the preoptic/lateral hypothalamic region.

The neocortical part of the brain is the cognitive part of the brain where sensory processing occurs. It is the neocortical pathway that enables us to perceive the scent of a rose and where past memories associated with the scent are immediately evoked.

The preoptic/lateral hypothalamic region is a noncognitive area that forms part of the 'limbic system'. This region enables us to associate the smell of rose with feelings of romance and a sense of relaxation. The limbic system was originally known as the rhinecephalon, or the 'smell brain'. Together with the hypothalamus the limbic system initiates and governs our emotions and instinctive drives such as sex, thirst and hunger.

One of the most important functions of the hypothalamus is the control of the autonomic nervous system, which regulates such functions as the heart rate, blood pressure, respiration, digestive activity and levels of hormones. Regulation of visceral functions depends on two systems. One is the sympathetic nervous system that prepares the body for fight or flight, raising the heart rate and the blood pressure — and decreasing digestive activity, since the blood flow is needed elsewhere. The parasympathetic nervous system does the reverse, preparing the body for more vegetative activities.

It is now possible to understand that the hypothalamus plays a very important role in regulating body functions and activities during times of stress, and that the essential oils via their influence on the limbic system and hypothalamus can play a very important role in the management of stress.

The Psychological Effects of Olfaction

Can the response of individuals to the aromas of essential oils be monitored, in the same way that the beating of the heart can be recorded? A traditional method that is used to measure psychological responses to odour is the use of psychometric scales in which the subject scales a list of descriptors relating to their psychological state/feelings. One of the problems with this technique is that the response is largely subjective.

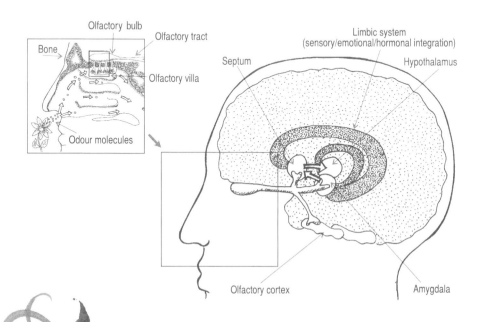

Olfactory pathway

36

A better method is to measure covert physiological responses that accompany behavioural changes. Long term psychophysiological changes can be measured using bodily fluids such as sweat, saliva, blood and urine. Short term changes can be measured by recording the minute bioelectrical potentials found throughout the body. These may include muscle potentials and heart rate as well as monitoring brainwave patterns generated within the brain. The latter is recorded by the electroencephalograph (EEG).

Techniques recording the electrical activity of the brain are non-invasive and rely on electrodes stuck or firmly held on to the scalp. The electrodes detect minute electrical currents on the surface of the brain and these electrical signals are then amplified by a factor of a million.

We are only just beginning to realise the significant influence that olfaction has on our behaviour, the way we feel and our emotions. One of the latest buzzwords is 'psycho-neuro-endocrino-immunology', which basically states that our mental and physical health is intrinsic.

Psychological stress causes a release of hormones such as adrenalin and cortisol, which suppress our immune defences, making us more susceptible to disease. Cortical reduces the level of T-helper cells and inhibits the production of natural killer (NK) cells. A depressed immune system will make the body more vulnerable to infection, which in turn leads to further emotional depression. Once this negative cycle of ill health begins, it can be difficult to break. The point that I am trying to make is that it is well established that certain essential oils, when inhaled can have a positive effect on one's mood, reducing stress levels, thus strengthening the immune system.

The role of the emotions has often been down played in our society, but this is beginning to change. It is now realised that the influence of emotion and mood is significant because, how you feel may determine what you think and ultimately how you behave.

Since the mind and body are intrinsically related, a change in the emotional or psychological disposition of an individual can have a dramatic result on their health as a whole. Since the limbic system, tagged the emotional 'control centre' of the brain, is especially susceptible to the effects of scents, it is possible to heighten or influence the underlying disposition or attitude of a person by subjecting them to certain odours.

For example, odours which carry a positive association can help to bring about a change of attitude, allowing the individual to re-experience pleasure and joy. Is there any way of qualifying and predicting an individual's emotional response to an odour?

While it is true to say that certain scents tend to produce specific physiological effects that are common to all people — e.g., lavender is relaxing while basil is stimulating — subjective psychological factors can override the more objective physiological response. It is difficult to make hard and fast rules about how an individual will react to a particular smell. This is because the effects of a given odour can be overridden by specific emotional associations and psychological preferences. Sometimes even an unpleasant smell can have beneficial results if the associations are positive. It is therefore not possible to assess accurately an individual's reaction to a particular odour without taking into account the following:

- How the odour was applied.
- How much was applied.
- The circumstances in which it was applied.
- The person to whom it was applied (e.g., age, sex).
- What mood the person was in when it was applied.
- What previous memory associations they may have with the odour.
- Cultural and social backgrounds.
- Anosmia or the inability to smell.
- Expectations or thoughts about the odour.

In conclusion, science and pharmacology have given us a glimpse into the miracles of the chemical complexity and the biodiversity of essential oils. It would however be wrong to reduce the essential oils to mere pharmacological compounds. We should embrace the diversity of the essential oils and to acknowledge that essential oils are so intricately involved with the chemistry of life. Their interactions are far too numerous to be even approximated by scientific inquiry. Scent has always transcended the material planes of consciousness and communicated directly with those of the soul.

The Essential Oils

There are hundreds of essential oils available for use. The fifty five essential oils listed here are generally easy to obtain and are commonly used in aromatherapy.

Aniseed

Aniseed oil is steam distilled from the seeds of *Pimpinella anisum*. Most of the aniseed oil available nowadays is actually distilled from *Illicum verum*, referred to as star anise. The two plants have the common name aniseed, but belong to totally different plant families. Both plants yield an essential oil which is chemically similar and which has similar properties.

Description
Aniseed oil is a clear to very pale yellow coloured oil with an intensely sweet clean odour, truly reminiscent of the crushed seeds. A very common description used is that of a 'liquorice-like odour'.

Uses
Aniseed oil is often used to flavour liquorice candy. It is well known for its calming effect on the digestive system. It assists in the relief of gastrointestinal disturbances such as colic and flatulence. Used in a vaporiser it helps to loosens and liquefies mucous and relieves symptoms of asthma, hay fever and sinusitis.

Methods of Application
Topical application — massage; Inhalation — direct inhalation, diffuser, oil vaporiser.

Safety
Aniseed oil is known to cause skin sensitisation in some individuals. In large doses it is reputed to have a neurotoxic effect.

Basil

Basil oil is steam distilled from the flowering tops and leaves of *Ocimum basilicum*. There are four principal chemotypes of basil. They are the methyl chavicol chemotype — which generally comes from the Comoro islands; the linalool chemotype — from France; the methyl cinnamate chemotype — from Haiti and Guatemala and the eugenol chemotype — from Russia, Egypt and Morocco.

Description
Sweet basil oil is a pale yellow or almost colourless liquid with a sweet-spicy, slightly green aroma.

Uses
Basil oil has an intensely fresh and vibrant aroma that will help relieve nervous tension, reduce anxiety and the stress of study or work. Used as an inhalation it clears the head, relieves intellectual fatigue and gives the mind strength and clarity. It is beneficial for the respiratory system and may be used for the relief of asthma, sinus congestion, bronchitis and influenza.

Methods of Application
Topical application — massage, ointment; Inhalation — direct inhalation, diffuser, oil vaporiser.

Safety
Basil oil may be sensitising in some individuals. It is best to avoid using basil oil during pregnancy.

Bay, Laurel

Bay oil is distilled from the leaves of *Laurus nobilis*. It should not be confused with West Indian Bay which is distilled from *Pimento racemosa*.

Description
Bay oil is a pale yellow to very pale olive-green or almost colourless liquid of a fresh, strong but sweet, camphoraceous, spicy odour.

Uses
Bay oil is a good antiseptic for the respiratory system. It is an excellent expectorant with mucolytic properties. Bay oil is recommended for the treatment of chronic bronchitis. It has been described as an excellent cerebral stimulator and nerve tonic. It has a pronounced effect on the digestive system and may be useful as an appetite stimulant. It expels wind, settles the stomach and has a tonic effect on the liver and kidneys.

Methods of Application
Topical application — massage, compress, bath, skin care; Inhalation — direct inhalation, diffuser, oil vaporiser.

Safety
Bay oil is generally regarded as safe. Frequent use of bay laurel oil on the skin over a long period of time (approximately 3 weeks) can result in sensitisation and irritations.

Bergamot

Bergamot derives its name from the small town of Bergamo in Italy, where it was originally cultivated. The oil is produced by cold expression from the fruit peel of *Citrus aurantium* subsp. bergamia, a citrus fruit grown it Italy. It is one of the most commonly used essential oils in perfumery and is the main ingredient in Earl Grey tea.

Description
Bergamot oil is a green or olive-green, liquid with a rich, sweet, fruity and citrus odour.

Uses
Bergamot's uplifting and refreshing aroma helps to dispel nervous tension, irritability, anxiety and frustration. It blends well with most essential oils. For all tense, anxious or depressed people, bergamot oil may be used in a massage oil, in a bath oil or in a vaporiser.

The antiseptic properties of bergamot make it ideal for treating acne and oily skin. Bergamot oil may be blended with tea tree and lavender, added to a carrier oil such as cold pressed jojoba oil and dabbed onto eruptions to relieve the symptoms of cold sores, eczema and dermatitis.

Methods of Application
Topical application — massage, compress, bath, sitz bath, douche, skin care; Inhalation — direct inhalation, diffuser, oil vaporiser.

Safety
Do not use bergamot oil on the skin before exposure to the sun, as it is a photosensitiser. It increases the skin's reaction to sunlight and makes it more likely to burn.

Black Pepper

Black pepper oil is distilled from the dried crushed seeds of *Piper nigrum*. Black pepper grows mainly in Indonesia, India and Malaysia.

Description
Black pepper oil is an almost clear to pale greenish coloured liquid with a fresh, dry-woody, warm-spicy odour reminiscent of dried black pepper.

Uses
Black pepper is a warming oil that can be used in massage to alleviate arthritis, muscular aches and fatigue. It may be used for the relief of indigestion, as it encourages peristalsis

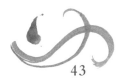

and is said to be useful for improving the tone of the colon muscles. In a vaporiser it may be used to promote confidence and focus.

Methods of Application
Topical application — massage, compress, ointment;
Inhalation — direct inhalation, diffuser, oil vaporiser.

Safety
Black pepper oil is non-toxic, non-irritating and non-sensitising.

Cajeput

Cajeput oil is steam distilled from the leaves and buds of *Melaleuca cajeputi*. The name of the oil is derived from the Malay word kayu-puti, a white tree which grows abundantly in Malaysia and the Molucca Islands.

Description
Cajeput oil is a colourless to pale yellow or greenish coloured liquid with a powerful fresh, eucalyptus-like, camphoraceous odour.

Uses
Cajeput oil may be used in a massage oil for the temporary relief of headaches, arthritis, rheumatism and muscular aches and pain. It can be used as an inhalation for the temporary relief of respiratory problems such as coughs and colds, flu, sinusitis and mucous congestion. It can be used in skin care for the treatment of oily and congested skin.

Methods of Application
Topical application — massage, compress, bath, ointment, skin care;
Inhalation — direct inhalation, diffuser, oil vaporiser, steam inhalation.

Safety
Cajeput oil is non-toxic and non-sensitising, however it may irritate the skin. Therefore it needs to be well diluted and never allowed to come into contact with mucous membranes.

Cardamom

Cardamom oil is produced by the steam distillation of the seeds of *Elettaria cardamomum*. The seeds are enclosed in husks and should not be removed from the almost odourless hulls until prior to distillation. Cardamom is a native to tropical Asia and is now cultivated in Sri Lanka, India, Guatemala and El Salvador.

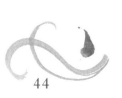

Description
Cardamom oil is an almost colourless or pale yellow liquid with a warm-spicy and slightly penetrating camphoraceous-cineole-like odour.

Uses
Cardamom oil is recommended for the treatment of digestive complaints such as colic, cramps, dyspepsia and flatulence. It can be used for catarrhal conditions of the respiratory system such as chronic bronchitis. Cardamom oil is a cephalic and a gentle tonic of the nervous system. Used in a vaporiser it is recommended for alleviating nervous exhaustion and depression.

Methods of Application
Topical application — massage, compress, bath;
Inhalation — direct inhalation, diffuser, oil vaporiser.

Safety
Cardamom oil is non-toxic, non-irritant and non-sensitising.

Carrot Seed

Carrot seed oil is steam distilled from the dried seed of *Daucus carota*. The essential oil is produced in France, Holland and Hungary. Carrot root oil is obtained by solvent extraction of the orange carrot root and it has a high concentration of carotenes.

Description
Carrot seed oil is a yellow or amber to pale orange-brown liquid with a tenacious, dry-woody somewhat earthy and spicy odour.

Uses
Carrot seed oil is well known for its detoxifying property. It may be used in a massage blend for the relief of arthritic and rheumatic pain. It assists in the treatment of fluid retention. It is also beneficial in skin care for damaged and aged skin.

Methods of Application
Topical application — massage, compress, bath, skin care;
Inhalation — direct inhalation, diffuser, oil vaporiser.

Safety
Carrot seed essential oil is non-toxic, non-irritant and non-sensitising.

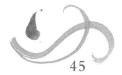

Cedarwood, Atlas

Atlas cedarwood oil is steam distilled from the wood of *Cedrus atlantica*. Atlas cedarwood is entirely different from Virginian cedarwood. It is believed to have originated from the famous Lebanon cedars which grow wild in Lebanon and on the island of Cyprus. These trees are now protected from being felled for essential oil distillation or lumber.

Description
Atlas cedarwood oil is a yellowish to orange-yellow or deep amber-coloured, viscous oil with a slightly camphoraceous top note and a sweet, tenacious woody undertone.

Uses
Atlas cedarwood oil may be used in a massage oil or vaporiser to help relieve nervous tension, stress and mild anxiety. Atlas cedarwood oil can be used in an inhalation to relieve symptoms of catarrh and temporarily relieve cough due to bronchial congestion. Atlas cedarwood oil is used in skin care for the maintenance of healthy hair and scalp.

Methods of Application
Topical application — massage, compress, bath, sitz bath, douche, skin care; Inhalation — direct inhalation, diffuser, oil vaporiser.

Safety
Atlas cedarwood oil is non-toxic, non-irritant and non-sensitising.

Cedarwood, Virginian

Virginian cedarwood oilis steam distilled from the wood of *Juniperus virginiana*. It is a slow growing evergreen tree with a narrow, dense and pyramidal crown. It grows in a fairly continuous belt running approximately from the central part of Virginia, through North Carolina and the northern edge of South Carolina, into Tennessee, central Kentucky and northern Alabama.

Description
Virginian cedarwood oil is a pale yellow to slightly orange-yellow coloured oil that is slightly less viscous than Atlas cedarwood oil. The odour is at first oily and woody with a sweet balsamic scent typical of cedarwood lumber.

Uses
It may be used in a massage oil or vaporiser to help relieve nervous tension, stress and mild anxiety. It relieves symptoms of catarrh and temporarily relieves cough due to bronchial

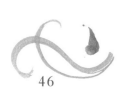

congestion. Virginian cedarwood oil is used in skin care for the maintenance of healthy hair and scalp.

Methods of Application
Topical application — massage, compress, bath, sitz bath, douche, skin care; Inhalation — direct inhalation, diffuser, oil vaporiser.

Safety
Virginian cedarwood oil is non-toxic, non-irritant and non-sensitising.

Chamomile, German

German chamomile oil is steam distilled from the dried flower heads of *Matricaria recutita*. It is also known as blue chamomile.

Description
German chamomile oil is a deep, inky blue somewhat viscous oil with an intensely sweet, herbaceous odour and a fresh fruity undertone.

Uses
German chamomile oil is rich in chamazulene, a sesquiterpene which gives the oil its beautiful blue colour and it's excellent anti-inflammatory and anti-allergenic properties. Many do not consider the strong medicinal and herbaceous aroma of German chamomile oil as pleasant when compared to Roman chamomile oil. However, when blended with lavender oil, which has similar properties, it takes on a soothing and calming aroma.

German chamomile oil is very valuable for many skin problems, especially when the skin is very sensitive, red or dry. It is beneficial in the treatment of eczema, urticaria and any dry, flaky and itchy skin conditions. German chamomile oil may be used in massage for the relief of muscular aches, inflamed joints and arthritic conditions.

German chamomile oil is particularly suitable for treating children. Rubbing a 1% dilution of German chamomile oil on the cheeks will help to alleviate teething pain.

Methods of Application
Topical application — massage, compress, ointment, bath, sitz bath, douche, skin care; Inhalation — direct inhalation, diffuser, oil vaporiser, steam inhalation.

Safety
German chamomile oil is non-toxic, non-irritant and non-sensitising.

Chamomile, Roman

Roman chamomile oil is distilled from the flowering tops of *Anthemis nobilis*. It is a pleasant smelling perennial with feathery fern-like leaves and branched stems of a creeping habit with daisy-like flowers. It is a native of Western Europe and is now cultivated in England, Belgium, France and Hungary.

Description
Roman chamomile oil is a pale yellow liquid with a sweet herbaceous, somewhat fruity-warm and tealeaf-like odour. The odour is extremely diffusive but it has little tenacity.

Uses
The main chemical constituents found in Roman chamomile oil are esters. Esters give the oil a pleasant, sweet herbaceous, somewhat fruity aroma and are responsible for giving Roman chamomile excellent antispasmodic and sedative properties. Roman chamomile oil is beneficial for relieving pain associated with irregular periods, PMS and for abdominal pain. Roman chamomile oil is also particularly helpful where stress and anxiety are inclined to make a person irritable or nervous. It is best combined with oils such as sandalwood, clary sage and lavender.

Methods of Application
Topical application — massage, compress, ointment, bath, sitz bath, douche, skin care; Inhalation — direct inhalation, diffuser, oil vaporiser.

Safety
Roman chamomile oil is non-toxic, non-irritant and generally non sensitising.

Cinnamon

Cinnamon is a bushy, evergreen tree up to 15m in height. The bark and leaves are strongly aromatic. Three distinct essential oils (bark, leaf and root) are produced from the cinnamon tree. Cinnamon is native to Sri Lanka, India and South East Asia. It has been introduced to the Seychelles, Zanzibar and Indonesia. Cinnamon bark essential oil is obtained by steam or water distillation of the bark of *Cinnamomum zeylanicum*.

Description
Cinnamon bark oil is a pale yellow to dark yellow or brownish yellow liquid with a extremely powerful, diffusive, warm-spicy and tenacious odour while cinnamon leaf oil is a yellow to brownish yellow liquid with a warm spicy, but rather harsh odour which lacks the rich body of the bark oil. Cinnamon leaf oil has some resemblance of the odour of clove leaf and clove stem oil.

Uses

Cinnamon bark oil is well known for its antimicrobial properties. However cinnamic aldehyde, its principle constituent is well known as a dermal sensitiser. Used in a vaporiser, the warm and spicy aroma of cinnamon bark helps to provide stamina and endurance.

Methods of Application

Inhalation — diffuser, oil vaporiser.

Safety

Cinnamon bark oil is a severe dermal irritant and sensitiser and is not recommended for topical application.

Citronella

Citronella oil is obtained from the steam distillation of the leaves of *Cymbopogon nardus,* which is cultivated in Sri Lanka or *Cymbopogon winterianus,* which is cultivated in Indonesia and the West Indies.

Description

C.nardus, commonly known as Ceylon citronella oil is a yellow to brownish yellow liquid with a distinctive warm-woody and yet fresh, grassy odour. *C.winterianus,* commonly known as Java citronella is a colourless to pale yellow liquid with sweet, fresh and lemony odour.

Uses

Citronella oil is well known for its ability to repel insects. The oil may also be used in skin care for combating excessive perspiration and oily skin.

Methods of Application

Topical application — massage, bath, skin care; Inhalation — direct inhalation, diffuser, oil vaporiser.

Safety

Citronella oil is non-toxic, non-irritant and non-sensitising. It may cause contact dermatitis in some individuals.

Clary Sage

Clary sage oil is distilled from the flowers and flowering tips of *Salvia sclarea,* a small shrub native of Southern Europe.

Description

Clary sage oil is a colourless to pale yellow or pale olive liquid with a sweet fruity, floral and herbaceous odour.

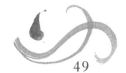

Uses

Clary sage oil is an excellent relaxant and is useful for alleviating nervousness, stress and anxiety. It is especially useful in a massage where there is muscular tension arising from mental and emotional stress. Clary sage oil is beneficial in treating asthma as it relaxes spasms in the bronchial tubes and relieves the anxiety and emotional tension experienced by asthma sufferers.

Clary sage is renowned for the relief it brings for menstrual cramps because of its antispasmodic properties. A warm compress of clary sage oil over the lower abdomen can be used to relieve menstrual cramping. It is also suggested that it may promote oestrogen secretion and is often recommended for oestrogen deficiency, PMS and dysmenorrhoea. It blends well with essential oils such as fennel, geranium and rose. Clary sage oil is an emmenagogue, and can help regulate scanty or missed periods. While it is best to avoid using clary sage oil during pregnancy, it can be used to encourage labour and to aid childbirth.

Methods of Application

Topical application — massage, compress, bath, skin care;
Inhalation — direct inhalation, diffuser, oil vaporiser.

Safety

Clary sage oil is non-toxic, non-irritant and non-sensitising.
The oil is contraindicated during pregnancy.

Clove Bud

Clove bud oil is obtained by water distillation from the dried flower buds of *Syzygium aromaticum*.

Description

Clove bud oil is a clear to yellow liquid, becoming brown with a strong, sweet and spicy odour.

Uses

Clove bud oil is well known for treating toothaches. A cotton bud is dipped in the undiluted oil and applied to the surface of the aching tooth and surrounding tissue, or if possible, inserted directly into the cavity where it will alleviate the pain for several hours.

The oil has excellent antiseptic properties. One percent emulsion of clove oil is said to have the antiseptic strength 3 to 4 times greater than phenol. Clove bud oil helps stimulate digestion, restores appetite and relieves flatulence. For rheumatic pains, clove oil will help relieve arthritis, rheumatism and sprains.

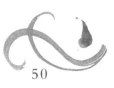

Used in a vaporiser the oil is considered a physical and mental tonic,
and should be used in conjunction with peppermint to ward of drowsiness.

Methods of Application
Topical application — massage, compress, ointment;
Inhalation — direct inhalation, diffuser, oil vaporiser.

Safety
Clove bud oil is a skin irritant and skin sensitiser.

Cypress

Cypress oil is steam distilled from the leaves and twigs of *Cypressus sempervirens.*

Description
Cypress oil is a pale yellow to almost colourless liquid with a sweet balsamic,
yet refreshing odour, reminiscent of pine needles and juniper berry oil.

Uses
Cypress oil is well known for assisting peripheral circulation and promoting
the health of capillaries. It should be blended with lemon and calendula infused
oil for the treatment of varicose veins. Use in a bath or massage oil to assist
in the treatment of fluid retention and applied topically it may be used
to alleviate the discomfort of haemorrhoids.

Methods of Application
Topical application — massage, compress, bath, skin care;
Inhalation — direct inhalation, diffuser, oil vaporiser.

Safety
Cypress oil has been reported to be generally non-toxic, non-irritant
and non-sensitising.

Eucalyptus

There are about 300 varieties of eucalyptus. The eucalyptus oils commonly
used in aromatherapy are distilled from the leaves of *Eucalyptus globulus,* known
as Blue Gum eucalyptus and from *Eucalyptus polybractea,* known as Blue Mallee
eucalyptus. Other species include *Eucalyptus citriodora* known as lemon scented
eucalyptus and *Eucalyptus dives* known as peppermint eucalyptus.

Description
Both *Eucalyptus globulus* and *Eucalyptus polybractea* have
a refreshing, slightly camphoraceous scent, typical of most
eucalyptus oils. *Eucalyptus citriodora* is a colourless to pale

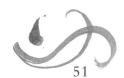

yellow liquid that has a strong and very fresh, citronella-like odour and *Eucalyptus dives* is colourless to pale yellow liquid that has a strong and very fresh, camphoraceous, spicy and minty odour.

Uses
The eucalyptus leaf oils are best known for their antiseptic and decongestant properties. They are ideal to use as an inhalation for the treatment of colds, catarrh and flu. They are beneficial for the treatment of sinusitis and are good for most throat infections, especially where there is a heavy discharge of mucous. For colds and flu, prepare a blend of 3 parts Blue Mallee eucalyptus oil, 3 parts lemon scented eucalyptus oil, 2 parts of thyme oil and 2 parts pine oil and use in an oil vaporiser or in a steam inhalation.

Eucalyptus has a pronounced cooling effect on the body, bringing an effective reduction of temperature. Dr Jean Valnet, a well-known French doctor who used essential oils, demonstrated the antiseptic properties of eucalyptus by spraying a solution containing 2% eucalyptus oil which was found to kill 70% of local airborne staphylococci.

All the eucalyptus leaf oils make excellent insect repellents. The oils should be blended with citronella oil and lavender oil to deter insects. The oils should be used in a vaporiser or a diluted blend applied topically.

Methods of Application
Topical application — massage, compress, bath, liniment, skin care; Inhalation — direct inhalation, diffuser, oil vaporiser, steam inhalation.

Safety
The eucalyptus leaf oils are non-toxic, non-irritant and non-sensitising. *Eucalyptus dives* is rich in piperitone, a ketone, which may be neurotoxic in high doses.

Everlasting

Everlasting oil is steam distilled from the flowering tops of *Helichrysum angustifolium*. When dried the brightly coloured, daisy-like flowers retain their colour and shape — hence the name *everlasting*. The plant grows wild and is cultivated in the south of France, Italy, former Yugoslavia and other Mediterranean countries.

Description
The oil is a pale yellow, oily liquid with a powerful and diffusive odour that is rather unique. It has a sweet-fruity and tea-like odour with an excellent tenacity.

Uses

Everlasting oil is well known for its ability to purify the blood. It stimulates the liver, gall bladder, kidneys, spleen and pancreas — the organs responsible for detoxifying the body.

Everlasting oil has analgesic and anti-inflammatory properties, making it beneficial for the treatment of rheumatoid arthritis. Its mucolytic, antispasmodic and expectorant properties makes it beneficial for treating sinus infections, bronchitis and coughs.

Everlasting oil is used in skin care because of its excellent anti-inflammatory properties and is recommended for the treatment of eczema and dermatitis.

Methods of Application

Topical application — massage, compress, bath, ointment, skin care; Inhalation — direct inhalation, diffuser, oil vaporiser.

Safety

Everlasting oil is non-toxic, non-irritant and non-sensitising.

Fennel

Fennel oil is steam distilled from the seeds of *Foeniculum vulgare*. It has a very sweet, fresh and slightly spicy smell reminiscent of aniseed.

Description

Fennel oil is a colourless to pale yellow liquid with a very sweet, but slightly earthy or peppery-spicy odour.

Uses

Fennel oil has long been used for the relief of indigestion and flatulence. Used in a massage oil it helps maintain healthy digestive function. Drinking a tea made from the seeds will provide quick relief from nausea, flatulence, indigestion, hiccups or colic.

Fennel oil is reputed to have an oestrogenic action, due to its main constituent anethole, which is an oestrogenic precursor. It helps to regularise the menstrual cycle, particularly when the periods are scanty and painful with cramping. It is also useful during menopause for reducing the unpleasant symptoms caused by fluctuating hormone levels.

When used in combination with juniper berry oil it is excellent for the treatment of cellulite and the accumulations of toxic wastes and fluid in the body.

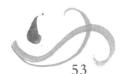

Methods of Application
Topical application — massage, compress, bath, skin care;
Inhalation — direct inhalation, diffuser, oil vaporiser.

Safety
Fennel oil should be used sparingly as it may be a skin irritant for people
with sensitive skin. Fennel oil should be avoided during pregnancy
and is not suitable for people suffering from epilepsy.

Frankincense

Frankincense oil is produced from the steam distillation of the resin
of various *Boswellia* species.

Description
Frankincense oil is a pale yellow or pale amber-greenish coloured liquid
with a strongly diffusive odour. It has a fresh, green-lemon odour.

Uses
Frankincense oil helps relieve nervous unrest and reduces the effects
of mild anxiety and nervous tension. It may be used for the temporary relief
of symptoms of coughs due to bronchial congestion. It is rejuvenating
and toning for mature skin and used in a vaporiser, it is spiritually uplifting
and soothing on the mind.

Methods of Application
Topical application — massage, compress, bath, liniment, skin care;
Inhalation — direct inhalation, diffuser, oil vaporiser, steam inhalation.

Safety
Frankincense oil is non-toxic, non-irritant and non-sensitising.

Geranium

Geranium oil is produced from the leaves of *Pelargonium graveolens.*
The finest quality geranium comes from the Reunion Islands and is known
as Bourbon geranium.

Description
Geranium oil is a beautiful pale green liquid and its aroma is described
as herbaceous and green, leafy with a subtle rosy note.

Uses
Geranium oil is well known for its balancing properties. It may
be used for alleviating stress, anxiety and depression. The oil

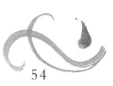

is recommended for correcting hormonal imbalances and mood swings associated with premenstrual syndrome and for reducing symptoms associated with menopause.

It may be used for treating cellulite and fluid retention. Geranium oil is useful in skin care for balancing sebum, the fatty secretion in the sebaceous glands. It is beneficial for sluggish, congested and oily skins.

Methods of Application
Topical application — massage, compress, bath, ointment, skin care;
Inhalation — direct inhalation, diffuser, oil vaporiser.

Safety
Geranium oil is non-toxic, non-irritant and non-sensitising. However, some cases of dermatitis in hypersensitive individuals caused by geranium oil have been documented.

Ginger

Ginger oil is produced by steam distillation of the dried, unpeeled, ground rhizomes of *Zingiber officinale*. Originally from India, ginger is now cultivated in India, China, most of South East Asia, Australia and the tropical regions of Africa.

Description
Ginger oil is a pale yellow to light amber coloured liquid. Its odour is warm, fresh, woody and spicy.

Uses
Ginger oil is considered a circulatory stimulant and tonic of the heart. It is recommended for poor circulation, cold hands and feet, cardiac fatigue and angina pectoris. The oil may be used in a compress or massage for rheumatism, arthritis and muscular pain of a cold contracting type.

Ginger oil stimulates and warms the digestive system. It is recommended for poor digestion, abdominal pain and flatulence. It should be blended with Roman chamomile oil and sweet orange oil to relieve travel and morning sickness. It is also recommended for catarrhal conditions, coughs, sinusitis and sore throats.

Methods of Application
Topical application — massage, compress, bath, ointment;
Inhalation — direct inhalation, diffuser, oil vaporiser.

Safety
Ginger oil is non-toxic and non-irritant. It may cause sensitisation in some individuals.

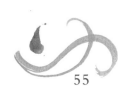

Grapefruit

Grapefruit oil is expressed from the peel of the fruit of *Citrus paradisi*.

Description
Grapefruit oil is yellowish to greenish yellow or pale orange liquid with a fresh citrus and sweet odour.

Uses
The properties of grapefruit oil are similar to that of lemon oil. Grapefruit oil is a lymphatic stimulant and is indicated for cellulitis, obesity and water retention. It has an uplifting and reviving effect which makes it valuable for treating stress, depression and nervous exhaustion. It is also beneficial in skin care for treating oily skin and acne.

Methods of Application
Topical application — massage, compress, bath, skin care;
Inhalation — direct inhalation, diffuser, oil vaporiser.

Safety
Grapefruit oil is non-toxic, non-irritating, non-sensitising and not phototoxic when used in normal dilution.

Jasmine, absolute

Jasmine absolute is obtained by solvent extraction from the flowers of *Jasminum grandiflorum*, cultivated in Egypt, Italy, Morocco and India.

Description
Jasmine absolute oil is a dark orange, somewhat viscous liquid with an intensely floral, warm, rich and highly diffusive odour.

Uses
The therapeutic value of jasmine oil is inseparable from the exquisite, comforting sweetness of its aroma, and the effect it has on the mind and emotions. Jasmine is considered one of the most effective essential oils for nervous anxiety, restlessness and depression.

Jasmine oil is one of the most useful oils to use during childbirth. If it is used as a massage oil on the abdomen and lower back in the early stages of labour it will relieve the pain and strengthen the contractions. It helps with the expulsion of the placenta after delivery and aids post natal recovery.

Methods of Application
Topical application — massage, compress, bath, skin care;
Inhalation — direct inhalation, diffuser, oil vaporiser, steam inhalation.

Safety
Jasmine absolute oil is non-toxic, non-irritating and non-sensitising.

Juniper

The best juniper oil is distilled from the berries of *Juniperus communis*.
An inferior oil is obtained from the leaves and twigs.

Description
Juniper berry oil is a clear to light yellow liquid with a fresh, yet warm sweet
pine-needle aroma.

Uses
Juniper berry oil is best known for its diuretic properties and may be used
in a massage oil or bath to treat fluid retention, cellulite, arthritis, gout
and rheumatic pain. The oil can be used for any skin condition which is slow
to heal, especially eczema that is weepy, dermatitis and psoriasis. The oil has
an astringent and detoxifying effect and may also be used to alleviate acne
and oily skin.

The cleansing and purifying properties of juniper works on the mental/
emotional level as well as the physical level. It is considered a psychologically
purifying oil.

Methods of Application
Topical application — massage, compress, bath, sitz bath, douche, skin care;
Inhalation — direct inhalation, diffuser, oil vaporiser.

Safety
Juniper berry oil is non-toxic, non-irritant and non-sensitising. Juniper oil
is contraindicated during pregnancy or for those with kidney disease.

Lavender

The English word lavender originally comes from the Latin verb 'lavare'
meaning 'to wash'. For centuries lavender has been used for soaps
and bath water. Lavender is perhaps the most widely used essential oil
not only for its therapeutic properties but also for its pleasant fragrance
in cosmetics, perfumery and craft works.

There are a variety of lavenders available, such as *Lavendula spica*, commonly
known as spike lavender; *Lavendula burnetii* commonly
known as lavandin; and the most commonly used lavender
in aromatherapy, *Lavendula officinalis* or *Lavendula
augustifolia*. The best quality lavender comes from the
alpine regions of France and from Tasmania.

Lavandin is produced from a hybrid of the true lavender and spike lavender. While the aroma of lavandin is not as refined as true lavender, it does have the same therapeutic properties but to a lesser degree.

Description
L.angustifolia oil is a colourless or pale yellow liquid of a sweet, floral herbaceous refreshing odour.

Uses
True lavender oil is refreshing and relaxing and for its calming, soothing and antiseptic properties. The oil calms the nerves and relaxes tension. It is used to relieve feelings of faintness, dizziness, headaches, nervous palpitations and insomnia. Lavender has a soothing effect on inflammation, hence its usefulness for burns, dermatitis, eczema, and psoriasis.

It is beneficial during childbirth, assisting in delivery and decreasing the severity of contractions. It helps to calm the mother and may be used as a refreshing compress for the head.

A lavender bath is refreshing, relaxing and therapeutic. It calms the emotions and makes a great evening bath for those with difficulty sleeping. A warm lavender bath or footbath is very good for relieving physical or nervous fatigue.

Methods of Application
Topical application — massage, compress, bath, sitz bath, douche, ointment, skin care; Inhalation — direct inhalation, diffuser, oil vaporiser, steam inhalation.

Safety
Lavender oil is non-toxic, non-irritating and non-sensitising.

Lavender, Spike

Spike lavender oil is steam distilled from the flowering tops of *Lavendula spica*.

Description
Spike lavender oil is a pale yellow to almost clear coloured liquid with a fresh camphoraceous and herbaceous odour and a somewhat dry-woody undertone.

Uses
Spike lavender oil contains a high percentage of cineole, also found in eucalyptus oil, camphor oil and rosemary oil. Spike lavender oil is useful as an inhalation for colds and respiratory infections, an insecticide and for the relief of muscular aches and pains.

Methods of Application
Topical application — massage, compress, bath, ointment, skin care;
Inhalation — direct inhalation, diffuser, oil vaporiser, steam inhalation.

Safety
Spike lavender oil is non-toxic, non-irritating and non-sensitising.

Lemon

Lemon oil is cold pressed from the peel of the ripe fruit of *Citrus limon*.

Description
Lemon oil is a yellow to greenish yellow or pale yellow liquid of a very light,
fresh and sweet odour, truly reminiscent of the ripe peel.

Uses
The fresh citrus scent of lemon is purifying and stimulating. It has been
described as a breath of fresh air on a hot summer's day. It encourages
awareness, clarity of thought and is emotionally invigorating.

Lemon oil is a bactericide, which is of great value for the treatment
of external wounds and infectious diseases. Lemon oil is also known
as an immunostimulant — that is the ability to stimulate the action
of the white blood cells.

Lemon oil is haemostatic, meaning that it helps stop bleeding. It improves
the function of the digestive system, counteracting acidity in the body.
Problems arising from too much acidity in the body give rise to painful
conditions such as rheumatism, gout and arthritis. Lemon has a toning effect
on the circulatory system and is especially appropriate in treating varicose veins.

Methods of Application
Topical application — massage, compress, bath, ointment, skin care;
Inhalation — direct inhalation, diffuser, oil vaporiser.

Safety
Lemon oil is non-toxic and non-irritanting, sensitisation
can occur in some people. It should not be used on the
skin prior to exposure to the sun as it is phototoxic.

Lemongrass

Lemongrass oil is steam distilled from fresh or partly dried leaves of *Cymbopogon citratus* or *Cymbopogon flexuosus.*

Description

Lemongrass oil is a yellow or amber coloured somewhat viscous liquid with a very strong, fresh, grassy, herbaceous and citrus odour.

Uses

The antiseptic property of lemongrass indicates that it would be excellent in a vaporiser to disinfect the air. It is considered a stimulant of the digestive system and is recommended for colitis, indigestion and gastroenteritis. The refreshing scent of lemongrass is uplifting and energising. It aids our logical thinking and is ideal to use at home or work or wherever clear, fresh thinking and good concentration is needed.

Lemongrass oil is referred to as the *'connective tissue oil'*. It tightens the elastin fibres in the epidermis and in the subcutis. The oil is recommended in the after-care of sports injuries, sprains, bruises and dislocations.

Methods of Application

Topical application — massage, compress, skin care;
Inhalation — direct inhalation, diffuser, oil vaporiser.

Safety

Lemongrass oil is non-toxic, however it may be irritating and sensitising in some individuals.

Lemon Myrtle

Lemon myrtle oil is steam distilled from the leaves of *Backhousia citriodora*, a tree native to southeast Queensland.

Description

Lemon myrtle oil is a yellow liquid with an intensive fresh, citrus aroma.

Uses

A refreshing and zesty citrus odour of lemon myrtle is reviving and uplifting. The oil may be useful for the temporary relief of headaches and muscular pain. Lemon myrtle helps to improve general well being.

Methods of Application

Topical application — massage, compress;
Inhalation — direct inhalation, diffuser, oil vaporiser.

Safety
Lemon myrtle oil is non-toxic, however it may be irritating and sensitising in some individuals.

Lime

There are two types of lime oil — distilled lime oil and cold pressed lime oil. Distilled lime oil is produced by steam distillation of the whole fruits or distilled the juice of the fruit of *Citrus medica*. Expressed lime oil is cold pressed from the fruit rind of green limes.

Limes are believed to have originated from northern India and adjacent areas of Burma. Limes were introduced to Persia, Palestine, Egypt, and Europe by the Arabs at about the same time as oranges and lemons.

Description
Distilled lime oil is a pale yellow to almost clear liquid with a fruity citrus odour. Cold pressed lime oil is a yellowish green to olive-green liquid with an intensely fresh citrus, rich and sweet odour.

Uses
The properties of cold pressed lime oil are similar to those of lemon oil. It has antimicrobial properties and is recommended for treating throat infections and influenza.

As with most citrus oils, lime oil is considered a digestive tonic and is recommended for digestive problems. Cold pressed lime oil is a lymphatic stimulant and may be used for the treatment of fluid retention and cellulite. Both cold pressed and distilled lime oil are refreshing and uplifting. They are ideal for fatigue and a tired mind, especially when there is apathy, anxiety and depression.

Methods of Application
Topical application — massage, compress, bath, skin care;
Inhalation — direct inhalation, diffuser, oil vaporiser.

Safety
Lime oil is non-toxic, non-irritating and non-sensitising. However cold pressed lime oil is phototoxic.

Mandarin

Mandarin oil is expressed from the fruit rind of *Citrus reticulata*. Mandarin is native to China and Indo-China and spread to other countries of the Far East where

it is extensively grown for domestic purposes. It was first introduced
to Europe in the eighteenth century.

Description
Mandarin oil is an orange-brown to dark yellowish-
brown or olive-brown coloured oil with an intensely sweet citrus odour.

Uses
The refreshing scent of mandarin oil with its cheerful aroma
is traditionally known in France as 'the children's remedy'. This is because
of its soothing qualities and affects of relieving colic and indigestion and
of maintaining a healthy digestive function. It helps to relieve insomnia,
nervous tension, stress and mild anxiety. Traditionally used to assist in the
treatment of fluid retention.

Mandarin oil is often used in combination with lavender oil, neroli oil and
wheatgerm oil to help prevent stretch marks during pregnancy.

Methods of Application
Topical application — massage, compress, bath, skin care;
Inhalation — direct inhalation, diffuser, oil vaporiser.

Safety
Mandarin oil is non-toxic, non-irritating and non-sensitising.

Manuka

Manuka is a small tree native to New Zealand. Most manuka is harvested
from wild plants as very little commercial cultivation is yet carried out.
There are several different Manuka chemotypes. The type with the
highest antimicrobial activity grows exclusively in the East Cape region
of New Zealand. Manuka oil is steam distilled from the leaves and twigs
of *Leptospermun scoparium*.

Description
Manuka oil is a clear yellow liquid with a distinctive spicy,
herbaceous and fresh aroma.

Uses
Manuka oil has been extensively used for generations in New Zealand
for its antimicrobial properties. The oil is recommended for the treatment
of ringworm, athletes foot, acne, skin eruptions, ulcers and wounds, cuts
and abrasions. It relieves muscular aches and pains, coughs, cold
and flu. It is reputed to have similar antibacterial properties
to *Melaleuca alternifolia*.

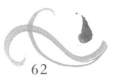

Methods of Application

Topical application — massage, compress, bath, sitz bath, douche, ointment, skin care; Inhalation — direct inhalation, diffuser, oil vaporiser, steam inhalation.

Safety

Manuka oil is non-toxic, non-irritating and non-sensitising.

Marjoram, sweet

Sweet marjoram oil is distilled from the flowering tops of *Majorana hortensis*, a native herb of the Mediterranean region.

Description

Sweet marjoram oil is a pale yellow or pale amber liquid with a warm-spicy, camphoraceous and woody odour.

Uses

Sweet marjoram oil is useful for relieving insomnia and reducing high blood pressure, especially when combined with lavender.

The warming effect of sweet marjoram makes it a useful oil in massage to relieve tired, tight and aching muscles, especially after heavy physical exertion and to reduce the pain of rheumatism and arthritis. Applied as a compress its analgesic and antispasmodic properties can offer relief from headaches and mild migraines.

Because sweet marjoram oil stimulates and strengthens intestinal peristalsis, it is a good digestive and carminative, relieving constipation, colic, flatulence and spasmodic indigestion. It has emmenagogue properties and may be used as a massage oil or compress over the lower abdomen to ease menstrual cramps.

Methods of Application

Topical application — massage, compress, bath, ointment, skin care; Inhalation — direct inhalation, diffuser, oil vaporiser, steam inhalation.

Safety

Sweet marjoram oil is non-toxic, non-irritating and non-sensitising.

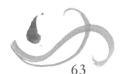

May Chang

May chang oil is steam distilled from the small, pepper-like fruits of *Litsea cubeba*.

Description
May chang oil is a pale yellow liquid with an intensely lemon-like, fresh, sweet aroma and a soft, sweet-fruity dryout.

Uses
May chang oil may be used as a treatment for coronary heart disease and high blood pressure. The pleasant refreshing citrus aroma of may chang can be used to alleviate stress and anxiety which may lead to depression. May chang oil is recommended for the treatment of oily skin and acne. It is also reputed to reduce excess perspiration and is a deodorant.

Methods of Application
Topical application — massage, compress, bath, skin care; Inhalation — direct inhalation, diffuser, oil vaporiser.

Safety
May chang oil is non-toxic, non-irritating and possibly sensitising in some individuals.

Myrrh

Myrrh is the resinous exudation, or gum, collected from the myrrh bush, botanically known as *Commiphora molmol*, either when it is wounded or from natural fissures. Myrrh oil is steam distillation from the myrrh resin.

Description
Myrrh oil is a pale yellow to pale orange coloured liquid. It has a warm-spicy odour with a sharp-balsamic, slightly medicinal top note.

Uses
Myrrh oil is well known for its antibacterial, antifungal and anti-inflammatory actions. The tincture can be used in the treatment of mouth, gum and throat infections. The oil can be incorporated into an ointment and is applied externally to treat haemorrhoids, bed sores and wounds.

Myrrh oil is used for the treatment of chronic wounds and ulcers. This is due to its antiseptic, astringent, anti-inflammatory and antiphlogistic properties. It is beneficial for mature skin, wounds that are slow to heal, and for weepy eczema and athletes foot. It heals cracked and chapped skin and can be added to skin care creams.

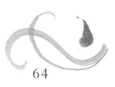

Myrrh oil instills a deep sense of calm and tranquility on the mind.
Myrrh oil is an excellent expectorant and as such is beneficial in the treatment
of coughs, bronchitis and colds. Myrrh oil is a uterine stimulant and promotes
menstruation thus relieving painful periods.

Methods of Application
Topical application — massage, compress, bath, ointment, skin care;
Inhalation — direct inhalation, diffuser, oil vaporiser.

Safety
Myrrh oil is non-toxic, non-irritating and non-sensitising.
It is contraindicated during pregnancy.

Myrtle

Myrtle oil is produced by steam distillation of the leaves
and twigs of *Myrtus communis.*

Description
Myrtle oil is a pale yellow to orange-yellow liquid with a fresh, camphoraceous,
spicy and herbaceous odour.

Uses
Myrtle oil is beneficial for chronic conditions of the respiratory system such
as bronchitis, catarrhal conditions and chronic coughs. It has an unobtrusive
odour and is well tolerated by young children. It is slightly sedative,
unlike eucalyptus oil which has a stimulating odour, and is recommended
as a chest rub or inhalation or oil burner at night.

Methods of Application
Topical application — massage, compress, bath, sitz bath, douche,
ointment, skin care; Inhalation — direct inhalation, diffuser,
oil vaporiser, steam inhalation.

Safety
Myrtle oil is non-toxic, non-irritating and non-sensitising.

Neroli

Neroli oil is obtained from the flowers of *Citrus aurantium* var. *amara,*
commonly known as the bitter orange tree. It is named after an Italian Princess,
Anna Maria de la Tremoille, Princess of Nerola, who used
neroli oil as her favourite perfume. While it is considered
expensive it is one of the most beautiful essential oils used
in aromatherapy.

Description
Neroli oil is a pale yellow oil which tends to become darker and more viscous with age. It has a powerful, light and refreshing floral top note with very little tenacity.

Uses
The light, refreshing and floral aroma of neroli oil has the ability to reduce stress and anxiety, and dispel depression. It has been described as being similar to the Bach Flower *Rescue Remedy*. It is beneficial for insomnia, particularly when the sleeplessness arises from anxiety. It is best used in a bath before bedtime. It is beneficial for the heart as it regulates heart rhythm and may help to reduce cramp-like nervous heart conditions such as palpitations.

Neroli oil is beneficial in skin care, for stimulating the growth of healthy new cells and for dry or sensitive skin.

Methods of Application
Topical application — massage, compress, bath, ointment, skin care; Inhalation — direct inhalation, diffuser, oil vaporiser.

Safety
Neroli oil is non-toxic, non-irritating and non-sensitising.

Nutmeg

Nutmeg oil is produced by steam distillation or steam and water distillation of dried nutmeg seeds from *Myristica fragrans*.

Description
Nutmeg oil is a pale yellow liquid with a light, fresh, warm-spicy and aromatic odour. The undertone and dryout remains warm and sweet with a slightly woody aroma.

Uses
Nutmeg oil may be used as a digestive stimulant. It is useful for the treatment of flatulence, nausea, chronic vomiting, and diarrhoea. It is an excellent oil to add to a massage oil because of its warming property for muscular aches and pains as well as rheumatism.

Methods of Application
Topical application — massage, compress, bath, ointment, skin care; Inhalation — direct inhalation, diffuser, oil vaporiser.

Safety
Nutmeg oil is non-toxic, non-irritating and non-sensitising.

Orange, sweet

Sweet orange oil is cold pressed from the outer peel
of the fruit of *Citrus sinensis*.

Description
Sweet orange oil is a rich yellow-orange to dark orange coloured liquid
with a fresh citrus odour, distinctly reminiscent of the odour of orange peel.

Uses
Sweet orange oil conveys a sense of warmth and joy. It is excellent for treating
insomnia, especially when combined with lavender oil or neroli oil. It blends with
most spice oils, especially clove and cinnamon oil, to create a wonderful spicy, zesty
and energising blend.

Sweet orange oil has a normalising effect on the peristaltic action of the
intestines. It is recommended for the treatment of constipation and chronic
diarrhoea. Sweet orange oil can be used in a massage oil to aid the body's
lymphatic system and may be used to relieve fluid retention caused
by accumulation of toxins.

Sweet orange oil is warming, harmonising and energising. It nourishes the soul
and feeds it with feelings of joy and happiness. Sweet orange oil is used in skin
care to treat dull and oily skin complexions.

Methods of Application
Topical application — massage, compress, bath, sitz bath, douche, ointment,
skin care; Inhalation — direct inhalation, diffuser, oil vaporiser,
steam inhalation.

Safety
Sweet orange oil is non-toxic, non-irritating and non-sensitising. Sweet orange
oil is not considered to be phototoxic, however bitter orange oil is phototoxic.

Palmarosa

Palmarosa is a tufted perennial grass with numerous stiff stems.
The grass grows wild in India, particularly northeast of Bombay
towards the Himalaya Mountains.

Palmarosa oil is steam distilled from wild growing, fresh or dried grass
of the plant *Cymbopogon martini*.

Description
Palmarosa oil is a pale yellow liquid with a sweet,
floral-rosy odour.

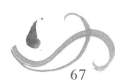

Uses
The sweet, refreshing rose-like fragrance of palmarosa oil is beneficial during times of stress. It helps to relieve nervous tension, stress and mild anxiety. Palmarosa oil is extensively used in skin care. It has excellent antiseptic and hydrating properties, helping to balance sebum production and is reputed to stimulate cellular regeneration.

Methods of Application
Topical application — massage, compress, bath, ointment, skin care; Inhalation — direct inhalation, diffuser, oil vaporiser.

Safety
Palmarosa oil is non-toxic, non-irritating and non-sensitising.

Patchouli

Patchouli is an aromatic, perennial shrub with erect stems, large green leaves and small white-pink flowers. Patchouli oil is steam distilled from the fermented leaves of *Pogostemom cablin*.

Description
Patchouli oil is a dark orange or brownish, viscous liquid with an extremely rich, sweet, herbaceous, aromatic, spicy and woody-balsamic odour.

Uses
The rich earthy scent of patchouli helps to relieve nervous tension and mild anxiety. It helps many skin problems and is used for the relief of symptoms of dermatitis and eczema. In skin care, patchouli oil may be used for dry, cracked or chapped skin.

Methods of Application
Topical application — massage, compress, bath, ointment, skin care; Inhalation — direct inhalation, diffuser, oil vaporiser.

Safety
Patchouli oil is non-toxic, non-irritating and non-sensitising.

Peppermint

Peppermint oil is steam distilled from the partially dried herb of *Mentha piperita*.

Description
Peppermint oil is a pale yellow or pale olive coloured liquid with a fresh, strong grassy-minty odour.

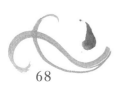

Uses

Peppermint oil is best known as a remedy for digestive upsets. It is valuable for colic, diarrhoea, indigestion, vomiting and stomach pain because of its antispasmodic action. It will relieve the contraction of smooth muscles of the stomach and intestines. Dilute well and massage the stomach and abdomen in a clockwise direction.

A cold compress of peppermint oil, or peppermint and lavender oil, applied to the forehead, back of the neck or temples will relieve headaches, and the pain of migraines, although not all migraine sufferers will tolerate the strong piercing scent of peppermint oil.

It may be used as an inhalant for asthma, bronchitis and sinus, and helps to clear stuffiness and headaches associated with colds. It is great in an oil burner to promote focus and assist in study as the fresh, vibrant scent of peppermint stimulates the brain and is said to promote clear thinking.

Methods of Application

Topical application — massage, compress, bath, ointment, skin care;
Inhalation — direct inhalation, diffuser, oil vaporiser, steam inhalation.

Safety

Peppermint oil is non-toxic, non-irritating and may occasionally be sensitising.

Pine

Pinus sylvestris oil is steam distilled from the needles, young branches and cones of the Scotch pine tree, which is widely grown all over Europe, the Baltic states, Russia, Central Europe and Southern European countries. The best quality *Pinus sylvestris* comes from Tryol, Austria.

Description

Pinus sylvestris oil is a clear liquid with a characteristic pine, fresh top note and a distinct sweetness.

Uses

Pine oil is regarded as a tonic to the lungs, kidneys and the nervous system. Pine oil is just as effective as rosemary and thyme for combating fatigue and nervous exhaustion.

Pine oil is recommended during times of convalescence or following an illness that leaves one feeling weak or with severe psychological stress.

It has excellent expectorant, balsamic and antiseptic properties, thus making it very useful for a wide variety of pulmonary complaints. It is one of the best oils to clear

cold phlegm from the lungs. It can be used for sinus and bronchial congestion, coughs, asthma and bronchitis.

Pine oil has a stimulating effect on the circulation and may be used in a liniment to relieve the pain of rheumatism and arthritis and for muscular aches from over exertion. Pine oil is also recommended for conditions such as cystitis and pyelitis.

Methods of Application
Topical application — massage, compress, bath, ointment, skin care; Inhalation — direct inhalation, diffuser, oil vaporiser, steam inhalation.

Safety
Pine oil is non-toxic, non-irritating and non-sensitising.

Rose

Rose oil is produced by solvent extraction or by distillation of the flowers of *Rosa centifolia* or *Rosa damascena*. Rose absolute oil is solvent extracted and is an orange-yellow coloured viscous oil with a rich, sweet, deep-rosy, tenacious odour. Rose otto oil, which is distilled, is a pale yellow coloured oil which tends to solidify into a translucent mass at temperatures below 20°C. Rose otto oil has a warm deep floral, slightly spicy and immensely rich rosy aroma.

Description
Rose absolute oil is a orange yellow to brown-orange viscous liquid with a sweet, deep-rosy, very tenacious odour. Rose otto oil is a pale yellow or slightly olive-yellow liquid which has a warm, deep-floral, slightly spicy and immensely rich odour with traces of a honey-like scent.

When cooled to a temperature of 20°C, rose otto oil separates into of white or colourless blades of crystals (stearopten), which when further cooled congeals to a translucent soft mass. When it is warmed with the heat of the hands, the oil will once again liquefy.

Uses
Rose is described as the queen of flowers. Rose oil is the most precious of all heavenly scents, refreshing the soul and bringing joy to the heart. Rose oil has been assigned to the heart and has a profound psychological effect. Most aromatherapists agree that rose oil is effective in all levels of life, for the soul, spirit and body. It is harmonising and anti-depressive, and may be used to help ease sorrow. It opens the heart and soothes feelings such as anger, fear and anxiety.

Rose oil has excellent softening and hydrating properties on the skin. Accompanied by its stimulating and antiseptic qualities, it is an ideal oil for all skin care, especially for mature, dry or sensitive skin. Rose oil can be used in an almond and calendula oil base for the treatment of broken capillaries, redness and inflammation of the skin.

Rose oil is extremely valuable for the treatment of gynaecological problems such as spasmodic and congestive dysmenorrhoea, uterine bleeding and functional infertility. The essential oil is very good at balancing women's hormone system. It strengthens the uterus, regulates menstruation, and relieves menstrual cramps.

Methods of Application
Topical application — massage, compress, bath, ointment, skin care; Inhalation — direct inhalation, diffuser, oil vaporiser.

Safety
Rose absolute and rose otto oil are non-toxic, non-irritating and non-sensitising.

Rosemary

Rosemary oil is distilled from the flowering tops and leaves of *Rosmarinus officinalis*. Greek philosophers wore garlands of rosemary to stimulate the mind and memory.

Description
Rosemary oil is a pale yellow to almost colourless liquid with a strong, fresh, woody-herbaceous aroma.

Uses
Rosemary is recommended for encouraging the flow of arterial blood and will benefit cardiac fatigue, palpitations, low blood pressure and cold hands and feet. As it increases blood flow to the brain, the oil can also be used for poor concentration and nervous debility.

The chemistry of the oil varies according to its country of origin and method of cultivation. Rosemary from Spain generally has a higher camphor content, rosemary from Tunisia tends to be higher in cineole and rosemary from France tends to contain verbenone. These variations are known as chemotypes.

The cineole chemotype is specific for lung and respiratory ailments, bronchitis, asthma and sinusitis. It makes a good painkiller and should be used for treating rheumatoid arthritis. When blended with peppermint or lavender oil it is an excellent treatment for preventing or easing the pain of headaches.

The verbenone chemotype is generally very expensive and it is used as a liver and gall bladder tonic. It helps to lower cholesterol levels in the blood. The camphor chemotype needs to be used with care because it contains a large proportion of ketones. It is the most specific heart tonic of all the essential oils of *Rosemarinus officinalis*. It is also an excellent oil for soothing rheumatic pain or cramps.

Rosemary oil is valuable for the maintenance of healthy hair and scalp.

Methods of Application
Topical application — massage, compress, bath, ointment, skin care; Inhalation — direct inhalation, diffuser, oil vaporiser.

Safety
Rosemary oil is non-toxic, non-irritating and non-sensitising. However it should not be used during pregnancy or by persons suffering from epilepsy. I would also suggest that individuals with high blood pressure avoid using rosemary oil.

Rosewood

Rosewood oil is steam distilled and occasionally water distilled from the chipped wood of *Aniba rosaeodora*.

Description
Rosewood oil is a colourless to pale yellow liquid with a refreshing, sweet-woody, somewhat floral-spicy odour.

Uses
Rosewood is often referred to as *Bois de Rose*. It has a distinctively sweet, woody, floral fragrance which is used for the temporary relief of headaches and to relieve nervous tension, stress and mild anxiety. It is a gentle oil that is ideally suited for general skin care use for all skin types - sensitive, dry, oily or mature. It is also recommended for the temporary relief of acne and dermatitis.

Methods of Application
Topical application — massage, compress, bath, ointment, skin care; Inhalation — direct inhalation, diffuser, oil vaporiser.

Safety
Rosewood oil is non-toxic, non-irritating and non-sensitising.

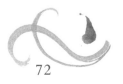

Sandalwood

Sandalwood oil is steam distilled or water distilled from the coarsely powdered wood and roots of *Santalum album*, a comparatively small tree which originates from India, Sri Lanka, Indonesia and surrounding islands.

Over the last five years we have seen the price of *Santalum album* oil increase. One of the major problems is that the demand for sandalwood is insatiable. Because of this demand, the Indian government has introduced strict controls to ensure the viable future of commercial supplies of the oil. In most states of India, the government now controls stock levels and all essential oil manufacturers must have a license. To manufacture the oil, only the heartwood of trees over 30 years old should be used. If younger trees are use, not only do you end up with an inferior oil, but the yield is considerably less.

Description
Sandalwood oil is a pale yellow to yellow viscous liquid having an extremely soft, sweet-woody and almost animal-balsamic odour, presenting little or no particular top note, and remaining uniform for a considerable length of time due to its outstanding tenacity.

Uses
Of all the essential oils, sandalwood has a long tradition of use in Eastern religious rites. Sandalwood's extremely soft, sweet and woody aroma promotes clarity of thought and induces a deep meditative state. It is an ideal remedy for nervous depression, fear, stress and a hectic daily tempo.

Sandalwood oil is indicated for conditions of a hot, inflammatory and catarrhal nature — particularly where the skin, intestines, genito-urinary system and lungs are involved. Applied to the skin, sandalwood oil is soothing, cooling and moisturising, and is primarily used for dry skin conditions caused by loss of moisture and skin inflammations. It may also be used to relieve both eczema and psoriasis. It is also beneficial for chronic dry coughs.

Methods of Application
Topical application — massage, compress, bath, sitz bath, douche, ointment, skin care; Inhalation — direct inhalation, diffuser, oil vaporiser, steam inhalation.

Safety
Sandalwood oil is non-toxic, non-irritating and non-sensitising.

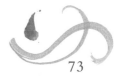

Spearmint

Spearmint oil is produced by steam distilled of the fresh flowering tops of *Mentha spicata*. Although it is a native to Europe, it is now common in North America and western Asia. The USA is the major producer of spearmint. Smaller quantities of spearmint oil are produced in Europe.

Description
Spearmint oil is a pale olive or pale yellow liquid with a warm, slightly green, herbaceous, penetrating odour reminiscent of the odour of the crushed herb.

Uses
Spearmint share similar properties to peppermint. It only has trace constituents of menthol so it is less harsh on the skin. This makes spearmint an excellent choice for children with digestive problems, such as nausea, flatulence, constipation and diarrhoea. Spearmint oil is recommended for indigestion and hepatobiliary disorders and it relieves flatulence, hiccups and nausea. Spearmint oil has an uplifting effect, reducing mental strain and fatigue, stress and depression. Used as an inhalation it can be used to decongest sinus problems, catarrhal conditions and asthma.

Methods of Application
Topical application — massage, compress, bath, ointment, skin care; Inhalation — direct inhalation, diffuser, oil vaporiser.

Safety
Spearmint oil is non-toxic, non-irritating and non-sensitising.

Tangerine

The botanical origin of tangerine and mandarin are similar. They are both considered to be varieties of the same species. The tangerine fruit is much larger than the mandarin, almost globoid, and its peel is usually yellow or pale yellow to reddish. Tangerine oil is cold pressed from the peel of the ripe fruit of *Citrus reticulata*.

Description
Tangerine oil is orange coloured, and with a fresh, sweet odour, reminiscent of bitter orange and sweet orange oil, rather than mandarin.

Uses
Tangerine oil has similar properties to mandarin and orange oil. It is a safe oil to use during pregnancy and is recommended in a massage blend to prevent stretch marks. For this purpose it should be blended with essential oils such as lavender and neroli and carrier oils such

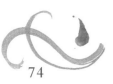

as wheatgerm and apricot kernel. It should be used daily from about the fifth month of pregnancy.

Tangerine has a tonic effect on the digestive system, and it may be used for calming the intestines and relieving flatulence. The oil is recommended in skin care for acne, congested and oily skin.

Methods of Application
Topical application — massage, compress, bath, sitz bath, douche, ointment, skin care; Inhalation — direct inhalation, diffuser, oil vaporiser, steam inhalation.

Safety
Tangerine oil is non-toxic, non-irritating and non-sensitising.

Tea Tree

Tea tree oil is distilled from the leaves of *Melaleuca alternifolia*, a native to the northern coast of New South Wales.

Description
Tea tree oil is a pale yellowish-green to almost clear coloured liquid with a warm, fresh, spicy-camphoraceous aroma.

Uses
This wonderful Australian oil should be compulsory in everyone's first aid kit. Tea tree has excellent antibacterial, antiviral and antifungal properties. It is known as an immuno-stimulant, so when the body is threatened with any infectious organism, tea tree oil will strengthen the body's immune system.

Tea tree oil is an ancient bush remedy for skin lesions or infected injuries. Liberally apply pure tea tree oil to the area and then dip a dressing in a 2.5% solution of oil in water, or pure oil, then bandage the wound. The dressing needs to be changed every 24 hours. This is suitable for any wound, skin abrasion, minor burn or weeping ulcer. Neat tea tree oil may be used to swab fungicidal outbreaks such as paronychia (nail infection), athlete's foot (tinea), vaginitis, thrush and cradle cap.

Ten drops in a tumbler of water may be used as a gargle to help clear throat infections, mouth ulcers or to eliminate bad breath. Used in a vaporiser the oil will be an excellent inhalation for congested nasal passages and respiratory infections. Tea tree oil blends well with lavender and bergamot oil for the treatment of acne.

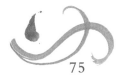

Methods of Application
Topical application — massage, compress, bath, sitz bath, douche, liniment, skin care; inhalation — direct inhalation, diffuser, oil vaporiser, steam inhalation.

Safety
Tea tree oil is non-toxic, non-irritating and possibly sensitising to some individuals.

Thyme

There are more than 300 different varieties of thyme. The most common species is *Thymus vulgaris*, known as garden or common or red thyme. Other species include *Thymus serpyllum*, known as creeping thyme or mother thyme; *Thymus zygis*, known as Spanish thyme; and *Thymus citrodorus*, known as lemon thyme.

Thyme oil is produced by water and steam distillation of the dried or partially dried leaves and flowering tops of thyme.

Description
Red thyme oil is a brownish-red, orange-red coloured liquid with an intense warm herbaceous odour that is somewhat spicy and distinctly aromatic.

Uses
Thyme oil is particularly effective for people who are fatigued, depressed or lethargic. It is very useful during convalescence and it stimulates the appetite. It helps to revive and strengthen both the body and mind and is reputed to stimulate the brain and improve memory. It stimulates circulation and may be used to raise low blood pressure.

Thyme oil is recommended for all infections. It stimulates the production of white blood corpuscles, so it strengthens the body's immune system. As a respiratory tonic, antiseptic, and expectorant, thyme may be used for any cold condition involving weakness, congestion and/or infection of the lungs. It will benefit chronic fatigue, shallow breathing, catarrhal coughs, and bronchitis, especially when there is copious amounts of clear or white catarrh.

According to Dr Jean Valnet an aqueous solution of 5% thyme kills typhus bacillus in 2 minutes. It can kill colon bacillus in 2–8 minutes, staphylococcus in 4–8 minutes and streptococcus and diphtheric bacillus in 4 minutes.

It is considered a nerve tonic and an intellectual and mental stimulant, which is beneficial in cases of nervous depression and mental fatigue. It is also recommended for headaches and stress related complaints.

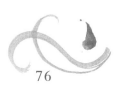

Thyme oil is used to ease gout, rheumatic pain and arthritis, and sporting injuries. It is especially useful when it is characterised by fixed pain of a contracted or cramping nature.

Methods of Application
Topical application — massage, compress, bath, liniment, skin care; Inhalation — direct inhalation, diffuser, oil vaporiser.

Safety
Thyme oil is non-toxic, non-irritating and a possible sensitiser in some individuals.

Vetiver

Vetiver oil is steam distilled from the roots of *Vetiveria zizanoides*. It is a tall densely tufted perennial grass which is native to India.

Description
Vetiver oil is an amber coloured to brownish viscous liquid with an odour that is sweet and very heavy, woody-earthy, reminiscent of the scent of roots and wet soil.

Uses
Vetiver oil has been described as deeply relaxing and is beneficial for anyone experiencing stress, anxiety, insomnia or depression. The oil is considered a classic for physical, mental and emotional burnout that can result from total exhaustion.

Vetiver oil is reputed to regulate hormonal secretions of oestrogen and progesterone. This makes vetiver an ideal oil to use during menopause, where both the hormones need supplementing. Its grounding and cooling effects will help to reduce the symptoms of hot flushes.

Methods of Application
Topical application — massage, compress, bath, ointment, skin care; Inhalation — direct inhalation, diffuser, oil vaporiser.

Safety
Vetiver oil is non-toxic, non-irritating and non-sensitising.

Ylang Ylang

This exquisite floral oil distilled from the flowers of *Cananga odorata* has a powerful, floral and intensely sweet aroma. The name ylang ylang means flower of flowers.

The finest quality ylang ylang comes from Madagascar. Ylang ylang is one of the few oils that is fractionally distilled. This means at several intervals during the distillation process, the oil is drawn off and sold separately as ylang extra, ylang 1st grade, 2nd grade and 3rd grade. This practice is obviously to the benefit of the perfume industry, which prefers the first fractions, as they possess a delicate floral aroma. For aromatherapy purposes I would recommend using ylang ylang extra, ylang ylang 1st grade or ylang ylang complete. Ylang ylang complete is usually a blend of ylang ylang extra, 1st grade and 2nd grade.

Description
Ylang ylang extra oil is a pale yellow oil with a powerful floral and intensely sweet odour. Ylang ylang complete oil is usually a yellowish, somewhat oily liquid with a powerful and intensely sweet, but soft balsamic floral odour with a floral woody undertone. Ylang ylang third grade oil is a yellowish oily liquid with a sweet-floral odour and balsamic-woody base note.

Uses
The rich floral scent of ylang ylang oil is euphoric, passionate, sensuous and uplifting. It is intensely charismatic and bewitching, and it creates feelings of peace and dispels anger. Like jasmine, rose and sandalwood oils, ylang ylang oil is known as an antidepressant, aphrodisiac and sedative. Used in a massage oil, vaporiser or bath it will help relieve nervous tension, stress, irritability and mild anxiety. Ylang ylang is known to slow down over-rapid breathing and over-rapid heart beat. These symptoms usually occur when someone is in shock, frightened or anxious, and sometimes when they are extremely angry.

Ylang ylang oil has a balancing effect on sebum production. This makes it suitable for both oily and dry skin types. It is used in hair care preparations to promote healthy hair.

Methods of Application
Topical application — massage, compress, bath, ointment, skin care;
Inhalation — direct inhalation, diffuser, oil vaporiser.

Safety
Ylang ylang oil is non-toxic, non-irritating and non-sensitising.
Excessive use may cause nausea or headaches.

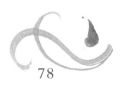

Carrier Oils

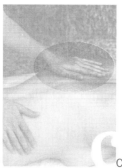

Cold-pressed vegetable oils are sometimes referred to as 'carrier' or 'base' oils and are commonly used for massage. These pure vegetable oils are not only highly nutritious, but they have many therapeutic properties when applied to the skin.

Carrier Oils

Carrier oils used in an aromatherapy massage should be cold pressed. Cold pressed oils are mechanically pressed from the seeds at low temperature, usually below 80°C. The oil is then filtered and bottled. This is the only method of preserving the original nutrients of the oils. The benefits of cold pressed oils that have been naturally extracted are that:

- they possess therapeutic properties.
- they enhance the absorption of essential oils into the skin.
- they are rich in fatty acids and other beneficial nutrients.

Unfortunately most commercially available oils have been extracted using high temperatures and chemicals, and are refined. This destroys and removes most of the natural nutrients of the vegetable oil.

Mineral derived oils should not be used in aromatherapy. Although the essential oils will dissolve in mineral oils, they have a very low penetration properties, so it reduces the essential oils ability to pass through the skin.

Almond, sweet

Sweet almond oil is extensively used in natural skin care preparations because of its moisturising properties. It is excellent for nourishing dried, tired, lifeless skin. It is a very good remedy for chafing, nappy rash, cradle cap and chapped skin.

Apricot Kernel

Apricot kernel oil is nourishing to the skin and hair, improving the elasticity of the skin. It is a light textured oil ideal for massage and cosmetic purposes. It makes a good base for the treatment of dry, mature, sensitive or inflamed skins.

Avocado

Avocado oil has traditionally been a popular skin care oil. This emerald green oil is rich in many nutrients, including vitamin A and D, lecithin and potassium. Avocado oil provides nourishment for the skin and is effective against dryness of the

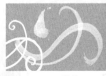

skin, eczema, sunburn and may be used for babies with nappy rash. The oil acts as a moisturising treatment for dry and mature skin types.

Evening Primrose

Evening primrose oil is rich in gamma linolenic acid (GLA), a very important essential fatty acid for regulating many bodily functions

The GLA found in evening primrose oil is biologically important as it affects much of the enzyme activity in our body. Every process that takes place in our body is triggered by the action of various enzymes, including the production of prostaglandins. Prostaglandins are responsible for:

- Lowering blood pressure
- Inhibiting thrombosis
- Inhibiting cholesterol
- Inhibiting inflammation
- Inhibiting platelet aggregation
- Regulating production of saliva and tears
- Regulating oestrogen, progestogen, and prolactin in the luteal phase of the menstrual cycle.

Prostaglandins are the end result of a chemical chain reaction that starts with essential fatty acids — notably linoleic acid, which is found in cold pressed oils. These essential fatty acids are not manufactured by the body, they can only be obtained from the diet.

A deficiency of these fatty acids may result in a wide range of disorders such as poor skin conditions, eczema type lesions, reproductive problems, circulatory problems, increased susceptibility to infection and poor wound healing.

Linoleic acid is converted into GLA, and then into diho-mogamma-linolenic acid and then to arachidonic acid. The latter two are present in all cell structures and are the precursors of prostaglandins. Research indicates that certain factors may inhibit the production of GLA. These include:

- A diet rich in saturated fats.
- A diet rich in processed vegetable oils.
  - Consumption of alcohol.
  - Diabetes.
  - The aging process.

- Lack of zinc, magnesium and vitamin B — all necessary for GLA formation.
- Viral infections, radiation, cancer.
- Stress.

It has been found that the GLA in evening primrose oil is a more efficient precursor of arachidonic acid than linoleic acid found in other vegetable oils.

As we know, GLA is essential to the formation of a number of compounds, the most important being PGE1. PGE1 assists in preventing thrombosis, lowering blood pressure and relieving angina pain. It reduces the production of cholesterol, enables insulin to work more effectively, prevents inflammation and controls arthritis. Now you can see why evening primrose oil works as panacea.

The elevated level of PGE2 is believed to be a major contributor to local inflammation and it now appears to be linked with lack of adequate amounts of PGE1. It therefore appears that aspirin and other steroid medications often given for rheumatoid arthritis are not the answer as they further lower PGE1 levels in the body. Instead we should be able to adjust the PGE1 levels through nutritional sources such as evening primrose oil.

Evening primrose oil can be used externally as a massage oil and has been found to be effective for the treatment of eczema and psoriasis, PMS, rheumatoid arthritis and weight reduction.

Jojoba

Pronounced *ho-ho-ba*. Jojoba oil is not susceptible to oxidation, it is highly bacteria resistant and will not turn rancid, so it has an extremely long shelf life. It is used extensively in cosmetics for this purpose and because it does not cause any allergic reactions, it is ideal for those with sensitive complexion, or oily and acne skin conditions that require delicate treatment.

Macadamia

Macadamia oil is high in palmitoleic acid, a mono-unsaturated fatty acid not commonly found in many other vegetable oils. Palmitoleic acid is also found in sebum, thus macadamia oil has often been recommended for older skin which starts to dry as sebum production diminishes. It is a highly nourishing and emollient oil and is recommended for dry and mature skin.

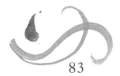

Neem

Neem oil is extracted from the seeds of *Azadirachta indica*. It is native to the Indian subcontinent. Neem has been used for centuries in India and is extensively used in Ayurvedic medicine to treat a multitude of ailments and conditions. Neem oil is used in soaps, shampoos and skin care preparations. It has antibacterial and antifungal properties and can be used for inhibiting viral and fungal infections such as warts, athlete's foot, ring worm, candida and staph.

Neem oil is also effective for the treatment of skin disorders such as rashes, eczema, scabies and ring worm. In skin care you can add neem oil to facial and body creams. In hair care preparations neem oil can be used in scalp preparations to prevent any itching and dandruff. It has been traditionally used as an effective head lice treatment.

It is used to repel house flies and fleas. Applied to the skin neem oil acts as an insect repellent as it keeps mosquitos, fleas and sand flies from biting.

Rosehip

Rosehip oil is extracted from the seeds of a rose bush which grows wild in the southern Andes. Extensive clinical research claims that rosehip oil is particularly beneficial in regenerative skin care. The oil is used to reduce wrinkles and signs of premature aging. It also helps to counteract the drying effects of the sun and also reduces the redness or hyperpigmentation of scars, reduces keloid scar tissue and loosens up fibrous chords.

It is believed that these important functions in the regeneration and repair of skin tissue are due to very high level of both linoleic and linolenic fatty acids (approximately 80%).

Sesame Seed

Sesame seed oil can be extracted from normal sesame seeds or seeds which have been roasted prior to being pressed. The latter oil is dark and smoky red and is often used in Asian cooking. The oil is rich in vitamin E and minerals calcium, magnesium and phosphorus. The oil is extensively used in Ayurveda medicine and can be used as a massage oil and in skin care preparations for its moisturising properties.

Soyabean

Cold pressed soyabean oil is the second highest source of natural vitamin E. It contains more lecithin than any other vegetable oil. The oil can be used as a massage oil and is suitable for all skin types.

Wheatgerm

Wheatgerm oil is an extremely valuable source of vitamin E and essential fatty acids. It is often used as an anti-oxidant. It promotes formation of new skin cells, improves circulation and assists in the healing of connective tissue.

Infused Oils

Infused oils are made by the traditional process of cold infusion, also known as maceration. Herbs are submerged in cold pressed vegetable oil and left to infuse. When complete, the oil is strained off, retaining the beneficial properties of the herb. They may be used as massage oils or for treating specific problems as outlined below.

Arnica

Arnica oil should be used for external applications only. It helps to temporarily relieve pain, reduce swelling, heals contusions and sprains, and disperse bruising. Arnica oil may be used as a compress and if applied immediately or as soon as possible to the injury it has astonishing healing qualities.

Calendula

Calendula oil's germicidal, anti-inflammatory, vulnerary and soothing properties make it ideal for the treatment cuts, grazes, abrasions, ulcers, skin inflammations, nappy rashes or cracked nipples. Calendula oil is soothing to rough and chapped skin, and may be used neat. It makes an excellent base oil for treating varicose veins and for dry eczema. In case of all venous inflammations, the oil should be lightly applied preferably blended with lemon and cypress essential oils. When applied consistently, calendula oil decreases the symptoms of varicose veins and venous congestion by inhibiting inflammation, toning tissue and promoting enhanced blood supply to tissue.

Carrot root

Carrot root oil is rich in beta-carotene and is used to promote healthy skin. Best used in a 10% dilution or less in wheatgerm oil for the treatment of dry, chapped and mature skin. This oil is bright orange and may stain clothing.

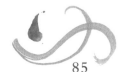

Hypericum

Hypericum is commonly known as St John's Wort. The oil is used topically for mild burns, bruises, sprains and wounds, especially where there is nerve tissue damage.

The oil assists the healing of wounds, has anti-inflammatory properties and is particularly soothing to inflamed nerves, making it helpful for the temporary relief of neuralgia, sciatica and rheumatic pain. It also assists in the healing of burns, bruises, haemorrhoids, varicose veins, wounds, sores and ulcers.

The oil is prepared by crushing the flowers and covering them in a fixed oil such as sweet almond, placing it in the sun for approximately three weeks. The oil is bright red and can be used externally for massage purposes to treat many of the conditions indicated.

A Guide to
Home Use

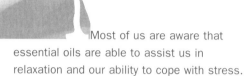

Most of us are aware that essential oils are able to assist us in relaxation and our ability to cope with stress.

However, many people are not aware that essential oils possess a much more diverse range of properties for treating a wide range of physiological and psychological conditions. Here we investigate the essential oils remarkable versatility and scope.

Aromatherapy First Aid

Bruises

Essential oils such as fennel, hyssop, rosemary and spike lavender are effective if applied to the area as soon as possible after bruising has occurred, preferably in an ice cold compress.

Arnica infused oil is a classic remedy for bruising and it can be applied neat to unbroken skin. In case of severe bruising such as that resulting from an accident, oils which stimulate the spleen such as black pepper, German chamomile and lavender will be helpful.

Burns

For minor burns follow the standard first aid procedure which involves applying running cold water over the burn until it has returned to normal body temperature. Lavender essential oil may then be applied, either a few drops in a bowl of water or a couple of drops neat. Apply at least three times a day. Never apply a lotion, ointment or vegetable oil to a burn.

Sunburn may be soothed by adding 5 drops of lavender and 2 drops of peppermint to a lukewarm bath and soaking in it for 10 minutes. Lavender and peppermint can also be added to fresh aloe vera gel and then applied to the sunburn to help soothe, heal and cool the burn.

Cuts, Wounds and Sores

For the treatment of cuts, wounds and sores the most beneficial essential oils are those with potent antiseptic properties. This includes essential oils such as eucalyptus, lavender, lemon, manuka and tea tree. Calendula infused oil can be used as a base oil as it is highly germicidal and a gentle antiseptic.

Be careful not to apply neat essential oils directly to open wounds as they may irritate the skin. You may dilute the essential oils in a castille soap base or in a dispersing bath oil base and dilute in water before applying to the skin.

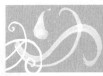

A typical antiseptic solution is:

tea tree	10 drops
lemon	5 drops
lavender	10 drops
dispersing bath oil	50ml

Add 5 ml of this solution to 100ml of warm water and wash the cut or wound.

Insect Bites and Repellents

A dab of neat tea tree or lavender essential oil on the affected area will help soothe and relieve the itching and stinging sensations, while reducing swelling. If the insect bite is swollen, apply a cold compress made with lavender oil.

Essential oils such as citronella, all eucalyptus oils, lavender, spike lavender, lemon myrtle, peppermint and tea tree may be used as insect repellents.

General Ailments

Arthritis

Arthritis is a disease of imbalanced body chemistry. Basically, the body is not eliminating uric acid efficiently. This may be caused by factors such as stress — which may reduce our body's ability to eliminate toxins or an incorrect diet; which gives the body more toxins to process.

In arthritis, uric acid is deposited as crystals in joint spaces causing inflammation, pain, stiffness, loss of mobility and eventually damage to the joints. The joints affected are often those which have been heavily used, as in sports, dance, and physically demanding jobs. Any site of early injury may become a vulnerable joint. In gout, a form of arthritis, the joints of the toes are most commonly affected. Gout attacks are intensely painful with acute inflammation of the joints. It is believed that rheumatoid arthritis may be caused by infection and that it is a form of auto-immune failure.

The accepted medical view is that arthritis is incurable and treatment is confined to the relief of pain by analgesics and anti-inflammatory drugs. Natural therapies aims at altering the body chemistry. Firstly, the toxic build up has to be eliminated, and then new accumulations of uric acid must be prevented. Circulation to the affected joints must be improved, to remove toxins and to improve the supply of nutrients to the affected area.

The essential oils can be used in a variety of ways to achieve these results. Detoxifying oils such as cypress, fennel, juniper and lemon can be used in a bath or massage into the affected area in a vegetable oil base.

Analgesic oils such as cajeput, black pepper, eucalyptus, ginger, lavender and rosemary can be used in a bath, local massage or compresses on the affected area. Local circulation can be improved by using essential oils such as black pepper, ginger and sweet marjoram. Whenever heat is applied to a stiff painful joint in the form of bath, hot compress or warming massage, it is important to move the joint as much as possible immediately afterwards, otherwise the heat can cause congestion, which makes the symptoms worse rather than better.

Gentle exercise is also recommended. Dietary advice is an important part of the effective overall treatment. A cleansing diet is recommended until pain and inflammation are reduced. This means eliminating red meat, coffee, tea, alcohol and refined foods.

If the arthritis is long standing it may not be possible to undo the extensive damage that has occurred to the joint surfaces, but in all cases pain can be reduced a great deal, mobility improved and further damage prevented.

Asthma

Asthma has typically been divided into two categories; extrinsic and intrinsic. Extrinsic or atopic asthma is closely linked with the presence of eczema, hay fever, urticaria and migraine.

Childhood asthma is often preceded for several months or even years by episodic coughing that later develops into a wheezy bronchitis and then eventually into asthma. Such children often have a history of slow recovery from upper respiratory tract viral infections. Environmental and/or dietary factors may also be important.

Intrinsic asthma is associated with a bronchial reaction that is not due to antigen-antibody stimulation, but rather to such factors as chemicals, cold air, exercise, infection or emotional upset.

Given the wide number of contributing factors the aromatherapy approach will need to be flexible and varied according to the immediate circumstances of the asthma sufferer. During a crisis, inhaling essential oils that have antispasmodic properties is the only practical help. This can be done by simply inhaling the essential oils from the bottle, or placing a few drops on a tissue or handkerchief.

Do not use steam inhalation as the heat from the steam will increase any inflammation of the mucous membranes and make the congestion even worse. Moisture, however, is helpful and a humidifier with a few drops of essential oil added is a good idea. Between attacks the entire thoracic area, back and chest should be massaged, with particular emphasis on techniques which open out the chest and shoulders. The selection of essential oils is dependent on whether an infection is present, and whether emotional factors are involved or if it is an allergic response.

Asthma's precipitated by infection (cold, flu, bronchitis, etc) with loose, copious mucus secretions is best treated with oils such as eucalyptus, myrtle, lemon and spike lavender. Asthma with viscid tenacious mucus is best treated with oils such as aniseed, cajeput, fennel, rosemary and peppermint. With allergies it is best to use oils such as everlasting, lavender and Roman chamomile. Another oil which has been found to be useful is frankincense. Not only is it used to treat the congestion, but it is also known to slow and deepen the breathing which is considered useful as a preventative measure in asthma.

Catarrh and Sinusitis

Catarrh, which is common to many respiratory problems, may be seen as the body's attempt to eliminate toxins via the mucous membranes. The most common causes of catarrh are colds, flu, hay fever, bronchitis, sinusitis and rhinitis. Diet plays an important part in many cases of catarrh. Dairy products are the most common culprit and should be excluded for a period by anyone who suffers catarrh frequently.

For immediate relief of congestion, a steam inhalation with essential oils is very effective. Essential oils that decongest and are expectorants, helping to clear the lungs and chest such as aniseed, cajeput, cedarwood, eucalyptus, fennel, frankincense, ginger, peppermint, pine, rosemary and thyme may be used.

Massage of the face, with special attention to the areas around the nose and over the sinuses will help to drain away excessive mucus. For catarrh caused by pollen and other irritants, anti-allergenic essential oils such as everlasting and German chamomile are the best choices.

Cellulite

Cellulite, the dimply fat layer seen mostly on the thighs and buttocks, is a concern of many women regardless of their age and weight. Cellulite is an accumulation of water and toxic wastes in the connective tissue surrounding fat cells, which in turn form nodules. It starts with a build up of toxins which in turn causes

the body to react by retaining fluid in an effort to flush out the toxins. All very well, except that the tissue around the fat cells tends to harden, imprisoning the fluid and causing unsightly bulges.

The main contributing factors to the development of cellulite are:

- Hormonal imbalance.
- Accumulation of wastes and toxins.
- Stress and emotional upheaval.
- Poor circulation.
- Unbalanced diet.
- Lack of correct exercises.
- Incorrect posture.

The main goals in eliminating cellulite are:

- To expel the body's toxins, wastes and impurities and improve the function of the body's eliminative and circulatory system.
- To strengthen the resistance and elasticity of the supporting connective tissues.

The combination of the correct diet, massage and use of essential oils, dry skin brushing as well as exercise means that cellulite can be completely eliminated.

Diet is important, because even if you manage to eliminate some cellulite using essential oils and massage, it will return unless you prevent it from reforming with a healthy diet. The anti-cellulite diet should cleanse and detoxify the body, enabling wastes to be eliminated. The anti-cellulite diet consists of eating only fresh natural foods. Natural herbal teas such as dandelion root, burdock and red clover are excellent as they are blood purifiers and assist the liver and kidneys in detoxification. Dry skin brushing is also important as it assists in the detoxification process.

The essential oils to select are detoxifying — stimulating to the liver, kidneys and lymphatic system; and hormonal balancing. The oils should be used in a massage and bath. The best type of massage is a lymphatic drainage massage.

The essential oils of cypress, juniper, fennel, grapefruit, geranium, rosemary and lemon are often used. The following formulas may be used:

Formula 1		Formula 2		Formula 3	
juniper	7 drops	fennel	3 drops	cypress	3 drops
rosemary	3 drops	cypress	5 drops	juniper	7 drops
lemon	5 drops	grapefruit	5 drops	lime	5 drops

The above formulae should be added to 30ml of vegetable oil or added to a bath. Use one formula for a week, then alternate the formula for the following week. Self massage of the cellulite areas using the essential oils is an excellent method. Use the massage oil as you would any body oil, after a bath or shower. Make sure that you use the oils twice a day for three to five weeks.

Exercise can be very effective to tone up your muscles, once you have managed to eliminate the worst cellulite. Although cellulite can be caused by a sedentary lifestyle, vigorous exercise alone will not make the slightest difference to the cellulite deposits that are already there. The best type of exercise is walking or swimming.

Reduce your stress levels, give yourself time to laugh and play, especially with the frantic pace we get caught up in. Try not to hold onto negative thoughts, as this is the only thing that prevents us from being truly healthy. Cellulite, according to Louise Hay in her well known book, *You Can Heal Your Life*, has much to do with holding onto childhood hurts, of not being wanted as a girl, or feeling hurt and resentful. Other causes include not resolving the emotional ups and downs in early life and holding onto resentments — especially towards your parents in early childhood.

Common Cold

Essential oils can play a vital role in reducing the discomfort of a cold or cough. They can be used as an inhalation or in a bath. A steam inhalation with the appropriate oils can combine several beneficial effects.

Desired Effect	Essential Oils Used
Expel mucus:	aniseed, Atlas cedarwood, cajeput, eucalyptus.
Clear the nasal passages:	peppermint, pine, eucalyptus, cajeput.
Soothe inflamed mucous membranes:	Atlas cedarwood, sandalwood, frankincense.
Antibacterial property:	cinnamon, eucalyptus, lemon, tea tree.
Stimulating the body's immune system:	eucalyptus, lavender, lemon, tea tree.
Reduce fever	peppermint, eucalyptus.
Warm the body	cinnamon, clove, ginger, black pepper.

Remember this should be included as part of a holistic treatment which may include warm herbal beverages such as peppermint, sage and yarrow. Some other tips to remember include:

- Maintain a high level of humidity especially if troubled by a croupy cough or difficult nasal breathing.
- Make sure you replace the fluids lost from coughing, sneezing and perspiring. Try to drink at least a glass of water every hour.
- Get plenty of rest.

Sore Throat

A sore throat can be caused by anything that irritates the sensitive mucous membranes at the back of the throat. Some irritants include viral and bacterial infections, allergic reactions, dust, smoke, fumes, extremely hot foods and drinks, tooth or gum infections and abrasions. Chronic coughing and excessively loud talking also irritates the throat. Typically, a sore throat is an extension of the common cold, tonsillitis, sinusitis or a viral infection.

Steam inhalations using essential oils such as lavender, tea tree, cajeput, manuka and myrtle will ease discomfort. A gentle massage to the throat and chest area with a massage oil blend containing frankincense, lavender and sandalwood can be used. These essential oils should also be used in a vaporiser, especially at night before going to bed. You may also add five drops of tea tree oil to a glass of warm water, mix well and gargle. Repeat two or three times a day. Continue until the condition has cleared up.

Indigestion

My first choice for any digestive upset is always peppermint. It is a digestive stimulant and carminative that will help

to relieve the discomforts of epigastric distention, from overeating and improper dietary habits. The antispasmodic and cholagogue properties of German chamomile, neroli, sweet orange and mandarin makes these essential oils useful in a variety of cases.

Other essential oils useful in the treatment of indigestion include ginger, rosemary, spearmint, Roman chamomile and cinnamon.

Hypertension

Hypertension is an important preventable cause of cardiovascular disease. Studies have shown that without treatment, hypertension greatly increases the incidence of cardiac failure, coronary heart diseases with angina pectoris, myocardial infarction, and renal failure. Arteriosclerosis and atherosclerosis are common precursors of hypertension because the arteries become obstructed with cholesterol plaque and the circulation of blood through the vessels becomes difficult.

While it will be necessary to make changes to the diet and lifestyle, aromatherapy can help to lower and stabilise blood pressure. There is also extensive clinical research that shows that regular massage effectively reduces high blood pressure.

The three main ways in which essential oils will help to alleviate hypertension are by;

- having a hypotensive effect.
- having a sedating and calming effect to reduce stress.
- having a detoxifying effect on the body.

The most important hypotensive essential oils are lavender, may chang, sweet marjoram and ylang ylang. While these essential oils may be used to lower high blood pressure, a selection of sedative, antidepressant and uplifting oils such as Roman chamomile, bergamot, neroli, rose and frankincense may also be used.

Detoxifying essential oils such as juniper berry and lemon are also recommended.

Essential oils such as rosemary, sage, hyssop and thyme are hypertensives and should not be used by anyone with high blood pressure.

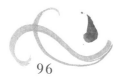

Muscular Aches and Pains

To treat muscular aches and pains resulting from overuse of the muscles, use analgesic and warming essential oils such as eucalyptus, ginger, sweet marjoram, rosemary or thyme.

Varicose Veins

The abnormal swelling of veins in the legs is a symptom of poor circulation and loss of elasticity in the walls of the veins, and particularly, in their valves. Aromatherapy is aimed at improving the general tone of the veins The most important oils for strengthening the veins are cypress, lemon and infused calendula oil. The following massage oil is effective in treating varicose veins.

cypress	10 drops
lemon	10 drops
geranium	5 drops
infused calendula oil	25ml
wheatgerm oil	25ml

Remember, varicose veins are usually due to inactivity, poor exercise or improper diet. Please consider an exercise program as well as using vitamin supplements such as vitamin E and C, especially one which has rutin and bioflavanoids.

Skin Conditions

Many skin problems are maninfestations of a deeper condition, such as an accumulation of toxins in the blood, hormonal imbalances, nervous tension or emotional upheavals. Essential oils are versatile as they are able to address these factors responsible for many of the skin condition in the first place.

Acne

Acne is commonly encountered in adolescence and pre-menstrually, but can proceed into adult life. Essential oils can be used to help clear the infection, regulate the amount of sebum produced, reduce inflammation and promote healing. The most beneficial oils are lavender, bergamot and tea tree, which are all bactericidal. Lavender is also soothing and healing and promotes the growth of healthy new cells. Bergamot is also an antidepressant and is useful for anyone with acne who is very self-conscious and may get depressed because of their condition.

Essential oils such as rosemary, lemon and geranium oils may also be used to help stimulate the lymphatic system to help clear the body of toxins. The following aromatherapy blend may be applied daily:

lemon	4 drops
lavender	4 drops
geranium	4 drops
tea tree	2 drops
apricot kernel oil	50 ml

It is also important to consider a holistic approach to acne by examining the diet and habits.

Cold Sores

Essential oils have been regularly used for the treatment of cold sores. Essential oils with antiviral properties that are used to treat cold sores include bergamot, eucalyptus, melissa and tea tree.

These oils should be applied very quickly at the first signs of eruption. Prepare these oils in an alcohol base by adding 6 drops of bergamot, eucalyptus and tea tree essential oils into 5mls of alcohol. Dab this blend on at first signs of onset and it will often help to prevent the blisters from developing.

Psoriasis

This condition results from a greatly increased turnover of epidermal cells. In people with psoriasis the new skin cells grow faster than the dead skin cells can be sloughed off, thus the skin appears red and thickened with a scaly appearance. Stress seems to play an important part in the onset of psoriasis, and the symptoms may come and go, as the individual is more or less relaxed.

Aromatherapy is valuable in reducing stress, a common trigger for psoriasis. Essential oils such as bergamot, lavender and sandalwood help to alleviate stress and anxiety. These oils may be used in an inhalation, massage or bath. Essential oils with anti-inflammatory properties such as lavender and German chamomile should be added to a base oil of jojoba, calendula infused and apricot kernel oil. You may also choose to use an emollient cream base that will reduce the scaliness and inflammation of the skin.

Cold pressed jojoba oil is an excellent base for massage. Research has found that jojoba applied to dry scalp and itchy skin problems such as psoriasis and eczema is very useful because of its emollient properties.

lavender	10 drops
bergamot	5 drops
juniper	5 drops
jojoba	25ml
apricot kernel oil	20ml
infused calendula oil	5ml

A holistic approach to psoriasis should also involve cleansing the body of toxins. This means strengthening the liver and stimulating the lymphatic system. Essential oils such as juniper berry or carrot seed can be used in a massage oil or bath. This should be combined with a diet of fresh, raw fruits and lightly cooked vegetables and wholegrain foods. Exclude alcohol, coffee, red meat and processed food with additives and sugars.

Stress Related Conditions

Stress is one of the major health problems in Western society today. It is responsible for at least 65% of our illnesses and any illness where stress is also present will be more difficult to treat. Conversely, when stress is relieved, it has been observed that treatment works better and recovery is faster.

Stress can be described as a person's reaction to a real or perceived threat, at a conscious or subconscious level, to his or her personal well being. The degree of harm a person suffers from the stress depends on their ability to cope with that threat.

It is important to realise that not all stress is bad, in fact a certain amount of stress is functional to maintaining optimal health. Hans Selye, often called 'The Father of Stress' referred to this optimal level as 'distress'. Should this level of distress be exceeded, causing dysfunction in the system, the person suffers 'stress'. An environment totally devoid of stress would therefore not be beneficial as some stress appears to be necessary for growth and change to take place and for the person to develop successful coping strategies.

It is very important that we recognise the first indications that something is wrong — mental tension, poor sleep, physical tension and lack of energy. Signs such as these may be part of everyday life for most of us and if we can cope with them adequately there is no reason for alarm. However, if we cannot cope with symptoms of stress we find that the symptoms become more chronic. These symptoms include:

• Tiredness, which develops into irritability, headaches and insomnia.

- Depression, anxiety, muscular pain, chronic aches, persistent infections, guilt, apathy, helplessness.
- Persecution complex, despair, increasing guilt and depression, susceptibility to viral infections. The body is really crying out for help. Unexplained pain, heart problems, strokes and high blood pressure may be experienced, along with all the other diseases that are thought to have their origin in stress such as ulcers.

Many essential oils are available to help cope with stress:

Essential oils to induce relaxation, reduce irritability, relieve headaches and overcome insomnia: *bergamot, Roman chamomile, clary sage, frankincense, lavender, petitgrain, rosewood, sweet marjoram, sweet orange, sandalwood, tangerine and ylang ylang.*

Essential oils to help relieve tiredness, aches and pain: *basil, black pepper, ginger, lemon, lime, geranium, rosemary, peppermint, pine, and thyme.*

Essential oils to help overcome depression, guilt, apathy, melancholy and feelings of helplessness: *bergamot, mandarin, melissa, neroli, rose and jasmine.*

Insomnia

The calming, soothing, balancing and anxiety reducing benefits of essential oils makes aromatherapy very effective for treating insomnia. Without a doubt the most commonly used essential oil for relieving insomnia is lavender. Extensive pharmacological studies and clinical trials have proven the benefits of lavender oil in treating insomnia.

Other useful essential oils include Roman chamomile, sweet marjoram, mandarin, neroli, sandalwood, petitgrain, sweet orange and ylang ylang. You can simply add a drop or two of any of these essential oils to your pillow or you may want to use these oils in a vaporiser, a warm bath before bedtime or in a massage oil.

Remember, if the problem persists, look at your lifestyle and attitude, and remove the stress factors that may be inducing the insomnia.

Mental Fatigue

When you feel exhausted from long periods of concentration use invigorating oils to help wake up the body and stimulate the mind and aid concentration. Essential oils such as basil, lemon,

peppermint, rosemary, ginger and lemongrass may be added to a vaporiser and used as an inhalation.

An alternative approach might be to use essential oils which will enhance sleep and are calming such as lavender, sweet marjoram, sandalwood and vetiver, thus ensuring someone suffering from fatigue gets adequate sleep to replenish their energy in a natural way.

Headaches

There are many oils that can be used to relieve headaches. One of the simplest techniques is to apply a drop of neat lavender to the temples and the back of the neck, to ease strain and tension. A cold compress of lavender or peppermint is also beneficial. For congested headaches due to blocked sinuses use a few drops of eucalyptus and peppermint as an inhalation either in an oil burner or a few drops on a tissue to inhale during the day. Other essential oils include Roman chamomile, clary sage, lemon, sweet marjoram, neroli and sandalwood. These oils are chosen for their soothing and relaxing properties.

When treating migraines, many people are often unable to tolerate the smell of essential oils or anyone touching their heads. Having said this, one of the most effective essential oils that I have come across for alleviating migraines is peppermint oil.

Depression

Depression is one of the most common human experiences. We may all experience it at some stage of our life or through those of our family and friends. We tend to think of depression as a natural response to the 'ups' and 'downs' of life. We are usually able to attribute depression to something specific, such as a death in the family, the loss of a job, a failure in love, feeling trapped or unproductive in one's life, or coping with a life-threatening or debilitating physical disease.

Many people will tend to deny that they have depression as there is often a social stigma attached to signs of 'mental illness' or not coping with life. When the cause is not obvious, we often identify basic attitudes or personality traits that may help to explain the depression reaction. We might decide, *'He has had a tough childhood and he's never got over it.'* or *'She has had a string of bad luck.'*

It is important to acknowledge depression as a very real illness that affects the entire mind and body. Depression can be a problem at any stage of life from childhood to adolescence, and throughout adulthood and old age.

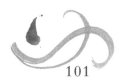

Aromatherapy can have a wonderful energising, uplifting effect on the nervous system and help to lift the spirits. When prescribing essential oils, care needs to be taken not to use a sedative oil if the depression is associated with fatigue or lethargy. On the other hand if depression is taking the form of restlessness, irritability and inability to sleep, such an oil would be ideal. Roman chamomile, German chamomile, clary sage, lavender, sandalwood and ylang ylang are essential oils that are both sedative and antidepressant. Oils such as bergamot, geranium, jasmine, neroli, tangerine, sweet orange and rose are antidepressant but at the same time uplifting.

When anxiety is associated with depression, neroli is considered one of the most valuable essential oils to use. Jasmine should always be considered to help boost one's self confidence.

Women, Pregnancy and Babies

Most women experience upsets in their menstrual cycle at some time during their life. This can usually be traced to some kind of hormonal imbalance. The type of symptoms that accompany such upsets are diverse and tend to affect the emotional and physical well being. Aromatherapy is considered one of the most effective methods of dealing with menstrual, pregnancy and menopausal concerns.

Menstrual Problems

Aromatherapy is ideally suited to relieve problems associated with menstruation. Probably the most commonly experienced problem is period pain and menstrual cramps, caused by spasm or contraction of the uterine muscles. A very gentle massage, a warm bath or compress with a hot water bottle over the abdomen with antispasmodic oils such as clary sage, lavender and Roman chamomile will effectively disperse the pain.

Any essential oil that is an emmenagogue is generally used for the treatment of amenorrhoea. Such essential oils include Roman chamomile, German chamomile, clary sage, fennel seed, lavender and sweet marjoram. Women whose menstrual flow is normal or heavy need to avoid these oils as they may cause the period to become very heavy. Obviously these oils will be useful in helping women whose periods are scanty or delayed. Remember that these oils should be avoided if there is any chance of being pregnant.

Women who suffer from abnormally heavy periods will find oils that have a regulating effect such as rose, geranium and cypress useful. Rose can be so beneficial for so many menstrual problems since it has a regulatory effect on the cycle and is a uterine tonic.

Pre-Menstrual Syndrome — PMS

Common symptoms associated with PMS are fatigue, headaches and bloating of the abdomen and legs. Breasts are often extremely tender and the skin may break out into acne. The blood sugar level may drop causing an insatiable craving for sugar.

PMS is usually caused by an imbalance in the ratio of the two female hormones, oestrogen and progesterone. These hormones are produced in much greater amounts throughout the latter two weeks of the menstrual cycle and have a profound influence on many bodily functions.

It has been found that the ratio of these two hormones in the blood stream has a strong regulatory effect on several of the chemical transmitter in the brain. This produces a state of anxiety and depression. Aromatherapy can be used to reduce depression and irritability, reduce fluid retention and relieve headaches. The following oils are ideal: bergamot, lavender, geranium, rose, juniper, cypress and rosemary.

The best base oil to use are those rich in essential fatty acids such as apricot kernel or sweet almond. Evening primrose oil is also found to be very beneficial and this may be applied externally as well as taking the capsules internally as a supplement.

The following is a useful recipe to use:

base oil	30ml
evening primrose oil	20ml
lavender	10 drops
juniper	10 drops
geranium	10 drops

Massage daily over the abdomen and hips starting from the last day of menstruation and continue until the next cycle.

Pregnancy

The popularity of aromatherapy during pregnancy has been mostly attributed to midwives willingness to incorporate natural and safe techniques to assist the birth process.

Pregnancy is a time of joy for most women and for the middle four or five months of a healthy pregnancy the mother has a look about her of glowing good health and she usually feels well and happy. During the early and late

months of many pregnancies, however and sometimes during the middle months also, a number of conditions related to the pregnancy can arise which cause varying degrees of discomfort or even distress.

The judicious use of essential oils together with appropriate forms of massage by a skilled therapist can help ease the discomforts of pregnancy and provide a sense of nurturing that will comfort the mother at times when she is likely to be feeling rather fragile. Aromatherapy is even more appropriate when the heightened sense of smell during pregnancy is taken into consideration.

The main cause of infant death is premature birth and the number one cause of premature birth is stress. There appears to be an epidemic of stress in much of the world today and it affects pregnant women at least as much as it does the rest of the population and possibly more. Caring use of aromatherapy treatments should help to reduce the stress felt by pregnant women and thereby possibly play a valuable role in reducing premature births caused by stress and the resulting prenatal deaths associated with it.

When considering essential oils during pregnancy we should first indicate a small group of essential oils which should not be used during pregnancy, either because they are toxic and can possibly harm the mother or the baby, or because of the risk of inducing miscarriage.

The oils which should be avoided include basil, clary sage, fennel, sweet marjoram, myrrh, pennyroyal, rosemary, sage, thyme and any other essential oil described as toxic.

Stretch Marks

An ideal recipe for stretch marks is:

lavender	1 drop
tangerine	1 drop
neroli	1 drop
apricot kernel oil	10 ml
wheatgerm oil	5 ml

It must be used daily from the fifth month of pregnancy to be really effective.

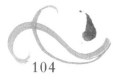

Morning Sickness

Morning sickness is a positive sign meaning that the placenta is sited. It often occurs in the morning, but can occur at any time of the day. It is believed to affect about 50% of women during the first three or four months of pregnancy. Four to five drops of ginger or spearmint essential oil may be used as an inhalation or used as a compress over the stomach. Alternatively, a few drops of the same oils on the pillowcase at night or inhaled from a tissue are helpful.

Labour

During labour, use 1% pure rose or jasmine oil in a base oil. Rose and jasmine are excellent uterine relaxants. A massage blend can be made using these essential oils.

Other essential oils which assist labour include clary sage, lavender and neroli. These essential oils may be used in a vaporiser or added to a bowl of warm water and left beside the bed, so that the vapours disperse into the air.

Menopause

Some women who stop menstruating in their 40's or 50's have little or no discomfort while others experience depression, irregular menstruation, excessively heavy periods, hot flushes, insomnia and a wide range of other symptoms for months or even years.

Many of the essential oils that help with menstrual irregularities earlier in life can be used to minimise the physical problems associated with menopause. Fennel, geranium and rose are essential oils that are particularly beneficial as hormone balancers. Other essential oils that are beneficial include Roman chamomile, bergamot, clary sage, jasmine, lavender and neroli.

Many women feel that they are losing their femininity. Rose can help to boost self confidence and one's femininity. Calcium supplements may be advisable, because as the production of oestrogen decreases, the bones become more brittle, leading to osteoporosis. This affects many post menopausal women, whose bones become fragile and fracture easily.

Babies

Babies, infants and children respond especially well to aromatherapy and massage. The dosage of essential oils for babies, infants and children is much lower than that used for adults.

Many studies have confirmed that babies who are massaged regularly feed and sleep better than those who are not. Colic and constipation are also reduced.

The dilution for a baby (0–12 months) should be less than 0.5%. This means adding no more than 5 drops of essential oil to 100ml of carrier oil. The oil can be applied every time the baby is bathed. Listed below are some of the common complaints that may be treated with aromatherapy.

Cradle cap:	Roman chamomile, lavender, neroli, calendula infused oil.
Colic:	Roman chamomile, neroli, mandarin.
Dry skin and eczema:	Roman chamomile, lavender, neroli, sandalwood.
Restlessness and insomnia:	Roman chamomile, lavender.
Nappy rash:	Calendula infused oil, German chamomile, lavender.
Teething pain:	Roman and German chamomile.

The massage should be very gentle and no pressure applied, especially to the top of the head where the fragile fontanelle is located. If the baby has eczema or nappy rash, Roman chamomile, lavender, sandalwood or neroli would be advisable. Unless you use a dispersing bath oil, it is not advisable to add essential oils to a bath for babies.

General Skin Care

The skin is the largest organ of the body and it performs many important tasks. The main functions of the skin include:

- maintaining body temperature.
- protecting the organs within our body from the environment, germs and damage.
- producing vitamin D.
- giving shape to the body structure.
- receiving stimuli from the environment.

Essential oils in general have a long tradition of use in skin care. The ancient Egyptians were probably the first to use essential oils in skin care.

Essential oils are ideal to utilise in skin care because they can be easily incorporated into creams, lotions, masks, ointments, gels, toners and perfumes.

The properties of essential oils that makes them beneficial
in skin care are:

- They are highly antiseptic.
- They help speed up the removal of old skin cells and stimulate the growth of new cells.
- They improve muscle tone and blood circulation.
- They help eliminate toxins.
- They reduce inflammation.
- They regulate sebum production.
- They reduce the impact of emotional stress.

Oily Skin

Excessive oiliness of the skin is caused by too much sebum being produced
in tiny glands just beneath the surface of the skin. Sebum is a natural lubricant
which everybody needs for the health and good appearance of the skin.
Essential oils can reduce the amount of sebum being produced and control
the acne-causing bacteria which thrive on the surface of oily skin.

Some people are puzzled by the idea of using oils to treat oily skin,
but of course the essential oils are non-greasy, and all traces of carrier oil should
be carefully removed after the treatment. My first choice of oils for an oily skin
is bergamot, lavender, geranium and palmarosa blended in equal proportions.
These oils can be blended in a base of jojoba oil. Bergamot and geranium have
a balancing effect on the sebaceous glands and lavender is very antiseptic and
will control bacteria on the surface of the skin.

Orange flower water, obtained by the distillation from the orange blossom
petals that are used to produce neroli oil, is also useful to use as a toner
for people with oily skin.

Dry Skin

The surface of the skin will appear dry. Treat dry skin with sweet almond,
apricot kernel, avocado and wheat germ and essential oils to gently stimulate
the sebaceous glands to function more efficiently.

Dry skin can be treated with German chamomile, jasmine,
sandalwood, neroli and rose essential oils. Lavender
and geranium have a balancing affect on the sebum
production and can also be beneficial.

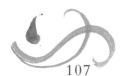

lavender	5 drops
sandalwood	5 drops
geranium	3 drops
jasmine	2 drops
apricot kernel oil	40ml
avocado oil	40ml
jojoba oil	10ml
wheatgerm oil	10ml

Mature Skin

The skin deteriorates with age in a number of ways. Apart from wrinkles, there may be discolouration, dryness, sagging and possibly thread veins in the cheeks. Aromatherapy treatment and lotions made with essential oils can help minimise all of these problems.

Most skins become less oily with age. To help restore the natural production of sebum, the natural oil which helps lubricate the skin, essential oils such as geranium, jasmine, neroli and rose can be used. It would be very useful to select rich carrier oils such as jojoba, avocado and a little wheatgerm oil.

Essential oil such as neroli and German chamomile stimulate the growth of new skin cells. Frankincense, palmarosa and rosewood can be used to help tone and rejuvenate dry and dull skin. Thread veins can be treated with German chamomile and rose, though it may take several months before real improvement is seen.

Regular massage with the essential oils can be beneficial as it stimulates local circulation. The massage should be done gently as vigorous massage on the already loose skin may make the problem worse. The following recipes may be used, a suitable base oil blend to use is as follows:

jojoba oil	20ml
avocado oil	10ml
rosehip oil	15ml
wheatgerm oil	5ml

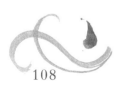

RECIPE 1		RECIPE 2	
palmarosa	3 drops	neroli	2 drops
fennel	2 drops	German chamomile	2 drops
frankincense	2 drops	lavender	3 drops
lavender	3 drops	rosewood	2 drops

The skin usually reflects the general health of the body, so ensure that you get enough exercise, proper nutrition, adequate sleep and avoid unnecessary pollutants.

110

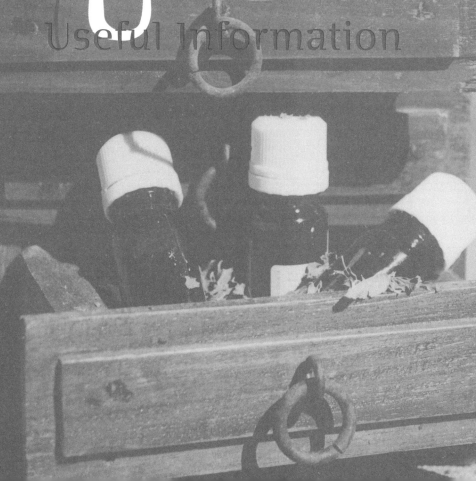

U

Useful Information

Aromatherapy Therapeutic Index

The following ailments cross reference list is only a suggested guide
to the aromatherapy treatment of common ailments. If in doubt please
seek the advice of a professionally trained aromatherapy practitioner.

Accumulated Toxins
carrot seed, fennel, geranium, grapefruit,
juniper berry, lemon, lime, sweet orange,
rosemary, tangerine

Aches and Pains
cajeput, clove bud, eucalyptus, ginger,
lavender, lemon myrtle, manuka,
nutmeg, peppermint, rosemary,
spike lavender, thyme

Acne
bergamot, geranium, grapefruit, lavender,
juniper berry, manuka, petitgrain,
rosewood, tangerine, tea tree

Aging Skin
carrot seed, carrot infused oil, frankincense,
lavender, myrrh, palmarosa, patchouli, rose
otto or absolute, rosehip oil, rosewood,
wheatgerm oil

Amenorrhoea
clary sage, fennel, geranium, juniper berry,
sweet marjoram, myrrh, rose

Anger
Roman chamomile, frankincense, geranium,
neroli, rose otto, sandalwood, ylang ylang

Anxiety
bergamot, Atlas or Virginian cedarwood,
frankincense, geranium, jasmine, lavender,
neroli, rose otto or absolute, rosewood,
ylang ylang

Asthma
cajeput, cypress, frankincense, eucalyptus,
lemon, lavender, Roman chamomile,
sweet marjoram, peppermint, pine,
rosemary, spearmint, thyme

Arthritis
black pepper, cajeput, carrot seed,
everlasting, lemon, German chamomile,
ginger, spike lavender, lavender,
juniper berry, sweet marjoram,
pine, rosemary, thyme

Blood Pressure, high
lavender, may chang, sweet marjoram,
ylang ylang

Blood Pressure, low
ginger, lemon, thyme, rosemary

Broken Capillaries
German chamomile, cypress,
geranium, rose

Bronchitis
aniseed, bay, cajeput, Atlas or Virginian
cedarwood, cardamon, everlasting,
eucalyptus, frankincense, lemon, myrthe,
myrrh, peppermnt, pine, rosemary,
sandalwood, thyme

Bruises
arnica infused oil, black pepper, fennel,
geranium, hypericum infused oil, lavender,
lemongrass, sweet marjoram

Burns
frankincense, lavender, everlasting, neroli,
tea tree

Catarrh

cajeput, Atlas or Virginian cedarwood, German chamomile, eucalyptus, frankincense, ginger, hyssop, spike lavender, sweet marjoram, peppermint, pine, tea tree, thyme

Cellulite

cypress, fennel, grapefruit, geranium, juniper berry, lemon, lime, rosemary, sweet orange

Chapped Skin

calendula infused oil, carrot infused oil, German chamomile, lavender, patchouli, sandalwood, sweet almond oil

Chilblains

black pepper, lavender, sweet marjoram, rosemary

Circulation, poor

black pepper, eucalyptus, ginger, lemon, marjoram, nutmeg, pine, rosemary, thyme

Colds and Flu

cajeput, cinnamon leaf or bark, eucalyptus, ginger, lavender, spike lavender, lemon, lime, manuka, myrrh, peppermint, pine, tea tree, thyme

Cold Sores

bergamot, German chamomile, lavender, manuka, tea tree

Colic

aniseed, German and Roman chamomile, fennel, ginger, lavender, sweet marjoram, peppermint

Congested skin

geranium, juniper berry, lavender, lemon

Constipation

black pepper, fennel, sweet marjoram, sweet orange, peppermint, spearmint

Coughs

aniseed, cajeput, Atlas or Virginian cedarwood, clary sage, eucalyptus, everlasting, frankincense, ginger, hyssop, spike lavender, manuka, myrrh, myrtle, pine, sandalwood, thyme

Cracked Skin

calendula infused oil, myrrh, patchouli

Cuts and Abrasions

calendula infused oil, carrot infused oil, lavender, lemon, manuka, tea tree

Dermatitis

bergamot, carrot seed, calendula infused oil, German and Roman chamomile, juniper berry, lavender, patchouli, rosewood, sandalwood

Dysmenorrhoea

clary sage, German and Roman chamomile, fennel, lavender, sweet marjoram, peppermint, rose

Eczema

bergamot, carrot seed, calendula infused oil, German and Roman chamomile, everlasting, juniper berry, lavender, myrrh, patchouli, sandalwood

Fever

eucalyptus, ginger, peppermint

Flatulence

bay, black pepper, cardamon, geranium, German and Roman chamomile, fennel, ginger, sweet majoram, lime, mandarin, nutmeg, orange, peppermint, spearmint, tangarine

Fluid Retention

carrot seed, cypress, fennel, geranium, grapefruit, juniper berry, lime, mandarin, sweet orange, rosemary, tangerine

Hayfever

cajeput, eucalyptus, peppermint, pine, tea tree

Headache
German and Roman chamomile,
eucalyptus, lavender, lemon myrtle,
sweet marjoram, peppermint, rosemary,
rosewood, thyme

Indigestion
black pepper, German and Roman
chamomile, fennel, ginger, lemongrass,
lime, sweet marjoram, mandarin, sweet
orange, peppermint, petitgrain, spearmint,
rosemary

Insomnia
Roman chamomile, lavender, sweet
marjoram, mandarin, neroli, sweet orange,
petitgrain, sandalwood, vetiver

Insect Repellent
basil, Atlas and Virginian cedarwood,
citronella, eucalyptus, geranium, lavender,
lemon myrtle, spike lavender, peppermint,
tea tree

Jet lag
peppermint, geranium, lemon

Mature skin
carrot seed, fennel, frankincense, lavender,
jasmine, mandarin, myrrh, neroli,
palmarosa, patchouli, rose, rosewood,
sandalwood

Menopause
cypress, fennel, geranium, lavender,
rose, vetiver

Menorrhagia
German and Roman chamomile,
cypress, rose

Menstrual Pain
German or Roman chamomile, clary sage,
lavender, sweet marjoram, rose

Muscular Aches and Pains
black pepper, cajeput, eucalyptus, ginger,
lavender, juniper berry, sweet marjoram,
nutmeg, peppermint, pine, rosemary, thyme

Nappy Rash
apricot kernel oil, avocado oil, calendula
infused oil, German chamomile, lavender,
jojoba oil, sweet almond oil, wheatgerm oil.

Nausea
black pepper, fennel, ginger, nutmeg,
peppermint, spearmint

Nervous Exhaustion
basil, cajeput, cardamom, cinnamon,
eucalyptus, ginger, grapefruit, lemongrass,
lemon, lime, may chang, peppermint, pine,
rosemary, spearmint, thyme, vetiver

Oily Skin
bergamot, cajeput, cypress, geranium,
grapefruit, juniper berry, lavender, lemon,
may chang, mandarin, myrtle, niaouli,
sweet orange, palmarosa, patchouli,
petitgrain, rosemary, tangerine, tea tree,
ylang ylang

Perspiration, Excessive
cypress, petitgrain

Pre Menstrual Tension
bergamot, German or Roman chamomile,
clary sage, evening primrose, geranium,
lavender, sweet marjoram, neroli, rose

Psoriasis
calendula infused oil, carrot seed,
German or Roman chamomile, everlasting,
evening primrose oil, jojoba oil, lavender,
myrrh, sandalwood

Rashes
calendula infused oil, German or Roman
chamomile, everlasting, hypericum infused
oil, lavender

Rheumatism
black pepper, cajeput, carrot seed, clove bud, German chamomile, everlasting, ginger, juniper berry, lavender, lemon, sweet marjoram, nutmeg, peppermint, pine, rosemary, thyme

Scars
frankincense, lavender, mandarin, neroli, sandalwood, tangerine

Sensitive skin
apricot kernel oil, calendula infused oil, German and Roman chamomile, evening primrose oil, everlasting, jojoba oil, lavender, neroli, sandalwood

Sinusitis
aniseed, cajeput, Atlas or Virginia cedarwood, everlasting, eucalyptus, ginger, niaouli, peppermint, pine, rosemary, spearmint, thyme.

Sprains
arnica infused oil, black pepper, cajeput, eucalyptus, nutmeg, sweet marjoram

Stress and Tension
basil, bergamot, Atlas or Virginian cedarwood, Roman chamomile, clary sage, frankincense, geranium, grapefruit, jasmine, lavender, mandarin, may chang, neroli, orange, palmarosa, patchouli, petitgrain, rose, rosewood, sandalwood, vetiver, ylang ylang

Sunburn
German chamomile, lavender, peppermint

Tinea
myrrh, patchouli, tea tree

Tired and Aching Muscles
black pepper, cajeput, ginger, spike lavender, lemongrass, lemon myrtle, manuka, sweet marjoram, pine, rosemary

Varicose Veins
lemon, cypress, calendula infused oil, geranium

Wounds
calendula infused oil, hypericum infused oil, everlasting, lavender, lemon, manuka, myrrh, tea tree

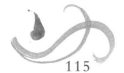

Resource Guide

Essential Oils

Perfect Potion

Perfect Potion carries an extensive range of pure therapeutic grade essential oils and carrier oils. It has also developed an extensive range of pure plant skin care products. Perfect Potion runs introductory workshops on aromatherapy, massage and making your own cosmetics. For your nearest Perfect Potion outlet or stockist please contact:

Perfect Potion
Unit 4, 90 Northlink Place
Virginia, QLD 4014
Ph: 07 3256 8500; Fax: 07 3256 8600; email: enquiries@perfectpotion.com.au
Website: www.perfectpotion.com.au

Aromatherapy Training

The International Centre of Holistic Aromatherapy

The International Centre of Holistic Aromatherapy offers an extensive range of aromatherapy courses, from Certificate III through to an Advanced Diploma of Aromatherapy. Training is accredited with the International Federation of Aromatherapists and the Australian government and is available by full time, part time or distance education. For more details please contact:

The International Centre of Holistic Aromatherapy
PO Box 635
Albert Street BC QLD 4002
Ph: 07 3012 8160; Fax: 07 3012 8161; email: info@icha.edu.au
Website: www.icha.edu.au

Professional Associations

The International Federation of Aromatherapists (IFA)

The IFA is a non-profit organisation dedicated to professional promotion of aromatherapy. Contact the IFA for a directory of accredited schools and practitioners. For more details contact:

IFA Australian Branch Inc
PO Box 786
Templestowe VIC 3106
Website: www.ifa.org.au

Journals

Aromatherapy Today

Aromatherapy Today is a journal for the professional aromatherapist. It is published quarterly. For more details contact:

Aromatherapy Today
PO Box 211
Kellyville NSW 2155
Website: www.aromatherapytoday.com

Glossary

Analgesic	Relieves pain.
Anti-allergenic	Reducing symptoms of allergy.
Antidepressant	Uplifting, counteracting melancholy.
Anti-inflammatory	Alleviates and reduces inflammation
Antiphlogistic	Alleviates and reduces inflammation
Antirheumatic	Helps relieve the pain of rheumatism.
Antiseptic	Helps to control infection.
Antispasmodic	Reducing spasms, relieves cramping.
Anti-sudorific	Reducing sweating.
Aphrodisiac	Exciting sexual desire.
Astringent	Contracts, tightens and binds tissue.
Bactericide	An agent that destroys bacteria.
Cardiac	Stimulating effect on the heart.
Carminative	Settles the digestive system, expulsion of gas from the intestines.
Cephalic	Stimulating and clearing the mind.
Cholagogue	Increases the secretion and flow of bile production into the duodenum.
Cicatrisant	Helps formation of scar tissue.
Cytophylactic	Encouraging growth of skin cells.
Decongestant	An agent which relieves or reduces, eg nasal mucous.
Deodorant	Destroying odour.
Depurative	Helps to purify the blood, detoxifying.
Digestive	A substance that aids the digestion of food.
Disinfectant	Prevents and combats the spread of germs.
Diuretic	Increases urine flow.
Emmenagogue	Promotes and regulates menstrual flow.
Expectorant	Helps to expel mucous from respiratory system.
Febrifuge	Cooling and reducing high body temperature.
Fungicide	Destroying fungal infections.
Galactagogue	Increasing production of milk.
Haemostatic	Arrests bleeding and haemorrhages.

Hepatic	Stimulates and aids function of liver and gall bladder.
Hypertensive	Increasing blood pressure.
Hypotensive	Lowering blood pressure.
Insecticide	Repelling insects.
Laxative	Aiding bowel evacuation.
Mucolytic	Dissolves or breaking down mucous.
Nervine	Strengthening or toning to the nerves or nervous system.
Parturient	Helping delivery in childbirth.
Prophylactic	Helping prevent disease.
Relaxant	Soothing, causing relaxation, relieving strain or tension.
Rubefacient	Warming and increasing blood flow.
Sedative	Reduces functional activity; calming.
Spasmolytic	Reducing spasms, relieves cramping.
Stimulant	Increases the physiological functions of the body.
Stomachic	Digestive aid and tonic, improves appetite.
Sudorific	Increases perspiration.
Tonic	Strengthens and improves bodily performance.
Uterine	Tonic to the uterus.
Vasoconstrictor	Contraction of blood vessel walls.
Vasodilator	Dilation of blood vessel walls.
Vermifuge	Expulsion of worms.
Vulnerary	Prevents tissue degeneration and arrests bleeding in wounds.

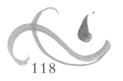

Recommended Reading and Bibliography

Battaglia S. *The complete guide to aromatherapy.* Perfect Potion, Brisbane, 1995.

Chapman J. *Aromatherapy — Recipes for your oil burner.* Harper Collins Publishers, Australia, 1998.

Chapman J. *More aromatherapy recipes from around the world.* Harper Collins Publishers, Australia, 2001

Davis P. *Aromatherapy A–Z,* 2nd ed., The C.W. Daniel Company Limited, United Kingdom, 1999.

Davis P. *Subtle aromatherapy.* The C.W. Daniel Company Limited, United Kingdom, 1991.

Fisher-Rizzi S. *Complete aromatherapy handbook.* Sterling Publishing Company, USA, 1990.

Hay L. *You can heal your life.* Specialist Publications, Australia, 1984.

Lawless J. *The encyclopedia of essential oils.* Element Books Limited, Great Britain, 1992.

Lavabre M. *Aromatherapy workbook.* Healing Art Press, USA. 1997.

Mojay G. *Aromatherapy for healing the spirit.* Hodder & Stoughton, United Kingdom, 1996.

Stubbin C. *Do it yourself pure plant skin care.* The International Centre of Holistic Aromatherapy, Australia, 1999.

Tisserand R, Balacs R. *Essential Oil Safety.* Churchill Livingstone, Great Britain, 1995.

Valnet J. *The practice of aromatherapy.* C.W. Daniel Company, Great Britain, 1980.

Worwood V. *The fragrant pharmacy.* MacMillam London Limited, England, 1990.

Worwood V. *The fragrant mind.* Doubleday, Great Britain, 1995.

Worwood V. *The fragrant spirit.* Doubleday, Great Britain, 1999.

Index